A Beginner's Guide to Critical Thinking and Writing in Health and Social Care

A Beginner's Guide to Critical Thinking and Writing in Health and Social Care

Third edition

Helen Aveyard and Marion Waite

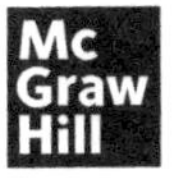

Open University Press

Open University Press
McGraw Hill
Unit 4
Foundation Park
Roxborough Way
Maidenhead
SL6 3UD

email: emea_uk_ireland@mheducation.com
world wide web: www.mheducation.co.uk

First published 2015
First published in this third edition 2024

Executive Editor: Sam Crowe
Editorial Assistant: Hannah Jones
Content Product Manager: Graham Jones

A catalogue record of this book is available from the British Library

ISBN-13: 9780335252534
ISBN-10: 0335252532
eISBN-13: 9780335252541

Typeset by Transforma Pvt. Ltd., Chennai, India

Praise for this book

of academic learning and professional reflection helps in developing confident, evidence aware, critical practitioners.

The level of detail in this text makes me feel quite superfluous to need! Learners can use this book independently to receive detailed, guided theory, linked to practical tasks. Each chapter contains various reflective and writing exercises with clear explanations related to expected responses. The chapter on demonstrating critical thinking skills in academic writing fully supports the academic skills teaching I am doing in the classroom and will be an excellent adjunct source."

Ruth Trout, Senior Lecturer in Acute Care, Programme and BSc Dissertation Lead, MSc Dissertation Supervisor, Buckinghamshire New University, UK

"This third edition of this book continues where the first and second editions excelled - in providing the foundations of critical thinking for students of health and social care. It strips away the mystery associated with 'being critical' and teaches that being critical is a skill that can be acquired.

Although aimed at pre-qualification students, it will also be valued by other students. It achieves its aims using a simple format and in language that is easy to understand. It is highly readable. It begins by demonstrating why critical thinking is a necessary aspect of professional practice. It then seeks to develop in students the habit of questioning normal practice and of searching for the best possible evidence to inform practice. It then guides students through the critical thinking skills of analysis, synthesis, and reflection.

It provides students with the tools and resources to develop these skills. The book then offers practical help in writing for assignments, and elsewhere, in ways which demonstrate critical thinking."

Dr David M Rea, School of Health and Social Care, Swansea University, UK

"A university educated healthcare workforce, be it through pre-registration programmes, or healthcare associate or apprenticeship routes, all have to regularly apply critical thinking

throughout their day-to-day professional practice and interactions, as is emphasised by this book by Aveyard and Waite. A prominent strength of the book is the link between critical thinking and evidence based practice, and another is the detailed guidance on the numerous ways in which to apply critical thinking to both academic writing and professional practice.

Learning to apply critical thinking is particularly relevant for both health profession students and for healthcare professionals returning to post-qualifying study, as it is for the substantial proportion of current healthcare professionals whose undergraduate education in other countries valued other models of education where critical thinking is not as strongly emphasised as it is in UK."

Neil Gopee RN, PhD, Lecturer in School of Health and Care,
Coventry University, UK

Contents

Acknowledgements   xiii

Introduction   xv

1   **What is 'critical thinking' and why is it important?**   1

Introduction to critical thinking: what it is and why it is
    important in health and social care   2
Defining critical thinking   5
Is critical thinking a new idea?   7
Critical thinking is not as common as you may think   9
An example of critical thinking in action   9
How you can think more critically – using our *'Six questions*
    for critical thinking'   12
The need to think critically has never been more important …   17
How critical thinking can help you in your professional
    practice and academic assignments   23
In summary   25
Key points   25

2   **Thinking more critically about readily available
information**   26

Critical thinking and the use of information/evidence   26
What types of information are readily available?   27
Thinking critically about the quality and usefulness of
    'readily available' information   28
In summary   41
Key points   42

3 Being more critical: finding the 'best available' evidence — 43

Why you need to dig deeper to find evidence — 44
Beginning the search process — 45
Using subject-specific electronic databases — 46
How you can plan and search for literature using specific databases — 49
What is the 'best available' evidence? — 55
Research evidence — 58
In summary — 75
Key points — 75

4 Demonstrating your critical thinking skills in your written work and presentations — 76

Why it is important to incorporate critical thinking into your writing and presentations — 77
When you need to incorporate critical thinking into your writing and presentations — 78
How you can develop good critical writing and presentations — 80
The importance of planning your work — 81
The importance of developing a clear, logical and thorough approach to your work — 86
Using different styles of writing and presenting — 92
An example of applying critical thinking skills to written academic work — 98
Demonstrating critical thinking in verbal presentations — 105
A checklist for assessing your critical thinking in written work and presentations — 107
In summary — 109
Key points — 109

5 Adopting critical thinking in your professional practice — 110

The professional context and complexity of critical thinking – connecting theory and practice — 111
How you can think critically about the influences on your professional practice: routine, relying on your experience, using professional judgement and learning from others — 113

Assessing and developing your skills as a critical thinker   122
Using questions to develop a more in-depth approach to
   critical thinking   136
Influencing the 'critical thinking' culture of your workplace   141
In summary   142
Key points   142

6   Shaping the future: what is the role of critical
    thinking in the development of health and social
    care services?   144

Why is critical thinking important for developing a
   broader perspective in your personal, professional and
   academic life?   145
What are the changes influencing health and social care in
   the twenty-first century, and how can critical thinking
   help you to respond to these?   148
How can you think more critically about these changes?   156
Skills and qualities needed to promote critical thinking in
   relation to broader perspectives in health and social care   158
Broadening your horizons in health and social care in your
   academic work and practice   160
In summary   170
Key points   170

Appendix: Useful websites   173

Glossary   176

References   181

Index   191

Acknowledgements

Thanks to Paul Aveyard and Chris Waite for support and for knowing when to leave us to it.

Thanks to Helen Baker for examples from learning disability nursing.

Thanks also to Jill Gregory for proof reading.

Introduction

This book is for you if you are:

- A student undertaking a pre-registration course in any of the health and social care professions.
- A registered practitioner, who may be returning to post-qualifying study after a career break.
- Working or studying anywhere in the world and want to develop your skills as a critical thinker and writer.

It is also for:

- Anyone who feels that they are not sure what to believe when they read conflicting professional information.
- Those who aspire to present information from different sources in their writing critically and concisely.
- Those who tend to take things at 'face value' and need to dig deeper into the evidence they come across.
- Practice assessors or mentors who are supporting students/learners in practice and are aware of the need to be more critical of the information and evidence they use. (The term 'practice assessor/mentor' will be used throughout to describe those who support learners in practice. A variety of other terms are used throughout the professions, including clinical educator, supervisor, practice educator/teacher, clinical tutor and instructor.)

You may already know that:

- There is a vast amount and many types of information available, and this is of variable quality.
- You need to be able to make sense of the information that you use in practice and present it effectively in your academic writing.

- Some findings from one source may conflict with those of another.
- You are legally and professionally accountable for your practice once you are a registered practitioner and need to use information appropriately.
- You cannot defend your practice by saying, 'I was told to do it this way'.

So ... where do you start?

You might feel unsure about where to begin when it comes to being critical of what you read, see or hear. Life would be easy if we could believe everything without the need to judge its quality. Furthermore, there is just so much information available. Making sense of the information and evidence you encounter can seem daunting.

This book will help you to understand and be more critical of the information you read, see or hear in a jargon-free way and guide you in presenting essential information logically.

Aim of the book

The aim of the book is to help you develop skills in critical thinking and writing – that is, not accepting everything you read, see and hear at face value but instead making sense of the information you use in your professional and/or university work. There is such a vast amount of information out there that, without these skills, it is difficult to know what to include in your academic assignments or how to incorporate new information into your practice. It is easy to feel overwhelmed and you may find that you make decisions in your professional practice or write academic assignments based on inappropriate evidence. As a result, poor decisions about professional practice are likely to be made, which can have a deep impact on patients and clients, and/or on the quality of your academic work. Critical thinking in writing and practice is therefore a vital skill that all students/learners and professionals need to develop from the very start of their practice experiences and in their academic work.

Furthermore, if you are a student, your ability to be critical will be assessed: a major component in almost all marking systems for those studying for professional qualifications in health and social care. In fact, 'being critical' is probably the key element of all higher education courses.

How to get the most from this book

- We recommend that you begin at the beginning and work through the book systematically, as the material is presented in the order in which we think it should be read.
- You can use the index if you have a particular topic or issue that you want to find out about.
- Use the glossary to find explanations of words you are unfamiliar with.
- Get access to the internet and gain confidence in searching using appropriate databases – don't leave it until you need to find information quickly.
- Be more critical of all of the sources of information you come across on a daily basis.
- Don't give up if you find something difficult or don't understand it.
- Feel good about every new thing that you have learned.
- You may find it helpful to work alongside a colleague or a fellow student/learner who is more confident in critical thinking in practice, to share your ideas and make sense of what you read as you progress through this book.

What's new in this edition?

We have responded to feedback on the second edition from a variety of readers and reviewers. Key changes we have made include the following:

- We have updated information sources where necessary, for example, incorporating up-to-date theory and new policy.
- We have included more examples to illustrate important points, such as adding more extracts demonstrating how you can write more critically.
- We have added more activities to help you to understand and engage with the ideas we discuss.
- We have incorporated advice about thinking and writing critically when you use online sources of information and social media, and about how such information may be used appropriately in health and social care practice and academic work.
- In response to evaluation from students, we have further developed our '**Six questions for critical thinking**' to make them clearer, more logical and easier to apply to academic work as well as practice issues.

Structure of the book

In the first chapter, we discuss the concept of critical thinking and why it is important. In Chapter 2, we consider the best response to 'readily available information'; by this, we mean information that you encounter on an everyday basis and do not need to look too hard for. In Chapter 3, we explore how you should 'dig a bit deeper' for evidence when you need to, using comprehensive search strategies. In Chapters 4 and 5, we discuss in more detail how to use critical thinking skills in your written academic work, presentations and practice, and introduce tools and methods to help you demonstrate critical thinking in your written work from note-taking to final draft. In Chapter 6, we consider the broader implications of critical thinking within health and social care.

We will use the following terms (alternatives may be used in your setting):

Health or social care professional: includes nurses, midwives, doctors, occupational therapists, physiotherapists, operating department practitioners, dieticians, paramedics, radiographers, speech and language therapists, art therapists, chiropodists/podiatrists, clinical scientists, orthoptists, prosthetists, social care workers, orthotists, osteopaths, pharmacists, health care scientists and dentists, plus members of any other disciplines registered with the Health and Care Professions Council or UK social work regulators.

Patient/client: used to refer to all service users that health and social care professionals may come into contact with. Although not stated, you may also need to consider carers' perspectives.

Practice assessor/mentor: used to describe those who support learners in practice.

Students/learners: used to refer to anyone, pre- or post-qualifying, undertaking study either formally or informally.

Examples

We have tried to include examples that may be easily understood by a range of professionals, as we all work within a wider team. We can learn a lot from the richness and diversity of examples from other professional groups even if they do not directly apply to our practice.

Web addresses

The web addresses we have provided were correct and accessible at the time of publication but do sometimes change. You may need to input the organization's details and search within their site if the address no longer works.

The symbols used in this book

Key information

Think point

Activity for you to do

1 What is 'critical thinking' and why is it important?

- *Introduction to critical thinking: what it is and why it is important in health and social care*
- *Defining critical thinking*
- *Is critical thinking a new idea?*
- *Critical thinking is not as common as you may think*
- *An example of critical thinking in action*
- *How you can think more critically – using our '**Six questions for critical thinking**'*
- *The need to think critically has never been more important …*
- *How critical thinking can help you in your professional practice and academic assignments*
- *In summary*
- *Key points*

In this chapter, we will:

- Introduce and define critical thinking and say why it is important.
- Give an example of critical thinking in action.

- Introduce our '**Six questions for critical thinking**'.
- Explore why critical thinking has become more important in recent years.
- Explore how critical thinking can help you in your academic assignments and professional decision-making.

Introduction to critical thinking: what it is and why it is important in health and social care

In short, critical thinking is about taking a step back and thinking logically and carefully about the information and evidence you have, rather than believing and acting on everything you read, see and hear. It is about seeking the best available evidence and using this to challenge your own assumptions and prior understanding. Critical thinking is about questioning and evaluating the information or evidence available to you. This is important because there is a lot of information and evidence available to inform your practice, much of which is of variable quality. You need to be able to make sense of it to ensure that you are acting on good quality information and evidence and therefore provide the optimum patient or client care.

Critical thinking is probably what you already do when you read a newspaper or watch a news item. You question what you read and often take what you read with a 'pinch of salt'. There is often good reason for this. Some newspapers and news stories are known for their shock tactics, including fake news, and it is generally wise not to believe everything you read. Critical thinking is probably also something you do when you listen to and take part in discussions about issues in your day-to-day life. You listen to others' thoughts, and probably join in, but inside you may wonder if there is any evidence behind the claims being made, such as whether claims about new skin care products or healthy foods are just a lot of 'hype'.

But maybe you aren't always critical of what you read, see and hear. Sometimes our own experiences make us biased and prevent us from being logical. To give an extreme example: someone who has just survived a plane crash is likely to perceive plane travel as dangerous, even though it is often quoted to be the safest form of travel. There are many times when we need to examine our perceptions and biases if we want to make logical choices.

You may have heard of the term **reflection**. We discuss this in more detail in Chapters 4 and 5 but, in principle, when you take the time to reflect, you consider more thoroughly your thoughts and feelings and how they impact on the decisions you make.

Consider what preconceived ideas and misconceptions about everyday life might affect what you think and do, and how you do it. 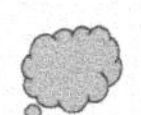

You might think that in professional life, everybody is rational – that professional life is tightly controlled. Yet health and social care professionals are individuals with different individual values, attitudes and beliefs that shape their approach to care delivery. In many ways, this is positive; we would not want to be looked after by robots or by people blindly following **guidelines** or instructions. However, it does leave room for different interpretations of how we should act in different situations, and different interpretations of information or evidence. This means that it is not wise to believe all you read, see and hear in a professional capacity. Even professional literature varies widely in quality, and it is essential that you can make sense of what you read. There is also a vast amount of information/evidence, some of it good and some less good. The quality of the dialogue you hear in professional practice will also vary.

The implications of this within health and social care are enormous. Rutter and Brown (2020) describe how false beliefs that we develop can lead to the making of wrong or badly judged decisions in practice. In other words, if we are not critical of the values, beliefs and attitudes we hold, this can lead to poor decision-making, and therefore impact negatively on our care. In our personal lives, it is ourselves who bear the consequences of this lack of critical thinking. In our professional lives, it is our patients and clients who will be affected if our care is based on false beliefs that lead to poor decision-making.

Imagine you experienced severe sickness many years ago when you were given the pain-killing drug morphine after an operation. You were intolerant of the drug – this is an extreme side effect that affects a very small proportion of people who are given morphine. Now, as a practitioner, you do not routinely offer morphine even though it is written up 'as required' and you try to dissuade people from consenting to it, even when they are in severe pain and morphine is the drug of choice.

or

Imagine you had a difficult experience after having your first baby and were not able to breastfeed. You were not given much encouragement or support and the advice you received was to bottle feed. Now, as a midwife, you are influenced by your early experiences and have very strong beliefs that all women should breastfeed and that it is your role to strongly encourage this.

or

Imagine you experienced severe bullying as a child at nursery. Now, as a social worker, you find yourself reluctant to advise parents to send their children to nursery even when your colleagues feel this is the most appropriate form of childcare.

All of these examples illustrate how a lack of critical thinking can lead to the delivery of inappropriate care. In each of these examples, previously held assumptions were not challenged, demonstrating how personal experiences and individual beliefs can lead to what may be badly judged professional decisions.

Kida (2006) provides a summary of the most common thinking errors. These include:

- being persuaded by *personal experience* rather than objective evidence; and
- preferring *evidence that supports our ideas* rather than objective evidence.

Rutter and Brown (2020) argue that critical thinking is about identifying and checking out our assumptions, looking at ideas and decisions from different perspectives, and taking informed action. Critical thinking, and in particular using reflection (as we discuss in Chapters 4 and 5), helps us to avoid these thinking errors. Critical thinking involves taking a step back and thinking logically about the evidence that you have.

Based on Facione's seminal work, we can see why critical thinking is important:

> *Critical thinking is essential as a tool of inquiry. As such, critical thinking is a liberating force in education and a powerful resource in one's personal and civic life. While not synonymous with good thinking, critical thinking is a pervasive and self-rectifying human phenomenon.*
>
> (1990: 2)

This is very important in health and social care. You cannot help bringing your own experiences with you into practice. What is important is that you acknowledge these and examine your beliefs in a critical way. You will hear a large amount of professional dialogue and have access to a vast amount of professional literature, and you need to work out what is useful and relevant and what is not; you need to make sure you are using reliable information or evidence wisely, both in your academic assignments and to inform your practice. In this book, we will explain how you can do this.

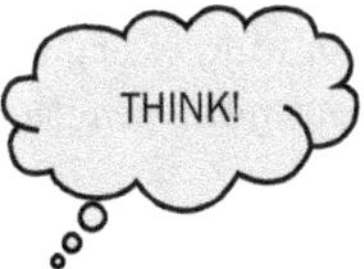

Figure 1.1

Defining critical thinking

There are many definitions of critical thinking, but if you look at them carefully, the message is largely consistent. Price and Harrington define critical thinking as:

> *a process where different information is gathered, sifted, synthesized and evaluated* … [which enables the professional to act] *as a knowledgeable doer – someone who selects, combines, judges and uses information in order to proceed in a professional manner.*
>
> (2019: 13)

Chatfield defines critical thinking as follows:

> [Critical thinking] *isn't about changing human nature, or pretending that we can or should act entirely rationally all the time. It's about learning to recognize our own – and others' – limitations; and knowing when to pause, think again and reach for the right questions in order to work out what is really going on.*
>
> (2018: 6)

Furthermore, Brookfield (2012) emphasizes how important it is to challenge one's own assumptions before engaging with additional information or evidence. In other words, if you are a critical thinker, you think carefully about what you read, see and hear. You also need to challenge your own previously held thoughts and assumptions. When you hear a news story or listen to a discussion among friends, you question the quality of the evidence and the conclusions drawn from that evidence. If the topic is important to you, you attempt to find out more information or evidence to help you make sense of the facts. This enables you to form an overall view and then apply it to the situation at hand.

To be a critical thinker means accessing the best available information and evidence to inform the decisions and judgements you make when delivering care. This means making every effort to search for good quality information/evidence about your practice. This is discussed in detail in Chapters 2 and 3.

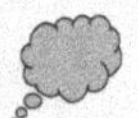

Have you been a critical thinker in the past?
Refer back to how you have used information in the past and consider the potential problems with your approach. Did you do any of the following?

- Believe what you were told without checking out the information/ evidence?
- Scan-read written information/evidence, rather than analyse it in depth?
- Use only readily available sources?
- Ignore **research** that didn't agree with your current practice?
- Listen to advice from colleagues without questioning?
- Copy practice/procedures that you observed without question?
- Believe everything that you read without questioning the authority of the writers or the quality of the arguments or evidence?

- Use only one or two sources?
- Select only sources that supported your view?

or

Do you feel that you fully consider the merits of each piece of information/evidence that you come across and seek out further resources or opinions when the available information does not seem to be complete?

We need to ensure that we consider all the facts before making judgements. This helps us personally and professionally to ensure we make considered and reflective decisions, considering the relevant evidence and not just following the advice and actions of others.

Is critical thinking a new idea?

Critical thinking is not a new idea in health and social care and many professionals have always questioned what they read, see and hear. The ancient roots of critical thinking date back to the ideas of the Greek philosopher Socrates, who is credited with pioneering a questioning and rational approach to problem-solving and encouraging people to reject statements made on the basis of confused meaning and inadequate evidence. We can see, then, that the concept of critical thinking has stood the test of time; however, as shown by **Examples 1** and **2** below, the concept is neither universally nor routinely applied.

Example 1: Evidence of a lack of critical thinking

Take, for example, the abundance of information that was circulating during the COVID-19 epidemic. Pertwee et al. (2022) refer to this as the 'info demic': where so much information is available, it is impossible to make sense of it. Pertwee and colleagues estimate that one tweet about COVID-19 was posted every 45 milliseconds! Many of these tweets contained speculation but had the effect of contributing to vaccine hesitancy and in some cases vaccine refusal. It is important to note that scares about health care and vaccinations in particular are nothing new (as described in **Example 2**) but the prevalence of speculation on social media reinforces the need to be critical of what you read.

Critical thinking requires that you look beyond the initial headline that catches your eye. In **Example 1**, cited above, critical thinking was required to question the sources of evidence and look wider and deeper at the reliable information that was published, such as that in academic journals.

Example 2: Further evidence of a lack of critical thinking

The controversy over the measles, mumps and rubella vaccination (MMR) provides another good example of why it is important to be critical of what you read, see and hear. The original research by Wakefield et al. (1998), which sparked a lack of confidence in the safety of the vaccine, was hugely influential.

This research paper has now been retracted by the publishing **journal**, *The Lancet.* This was done because the evidence presented was at a later date found to be flawed. However, before it was retracted, the paper attracted wide publicity. The authors of the paper described how 12 children who had received the MMR vaccination went on to develop either autism or bowel disease. Yet millions of children have had the MMR vaccination and suffered no ill effects. Also, children who have not been given the MMR vaccination have developed autism and/or bowel disease.

Anyone looking critically at this research can see that the evidence provided is not strong; in fact, it is very weak indeed and, as in **Example 1**, critical thinking is required to consider the method by which the data about the vaccination was collected and presented. A critical thinker would have used rational judgement and critical appraisal to explore the quality of the paper and to expose its weaknesses. Yet somehow the paper was not properly evaluated, and was so well publicized that vaccination rates plummeted as parents feared for the safety of the vaccination. In a further twist to this story, not only was the study very weak – and indeed, subsequent systematic reviews have found no link between autism/bowel disease and the MMR vaccination (Demicheli et al. 2012) – but much later on it was found to be fraudulent, in that there is evidence that the details of some of the 12 children described in the study were fabricated (Deer 2011).

Critical thinking is not as common as you may think

Having read **Examples 1** and **2**, you may not be surprised to read that we believe that critical thinking is not as common as one would like to think (which is why we have written this book). We have given the examples of misleading media headlines and a misinterpreted poor quality **research study**. Indeed, there is evidence that many professionals do not always think critically about the evidence they use. When Simone et al. (2012) reviewed the role of health care professionals in informing children and their parents about the MMR vaccination, they found that a minority of the professionals continued to hold negative attitudes about the vaccination because of Wakefield and colleagues' research. This suggests that these health care professionals had neither read nor thought critically about the evidence relating to this aspect of their practice.

Unfortunately, there are many other such examples. On his 'Bad Science' website [www.badscience.net] and in his book, Goldacre (2009) illustrates what can happen when people are not critical of information/ evidence that is presented to them. He explores many commonly held ideas about popular culture, most of which relate to health and social care. Using a critical approach, Goldacre examines the minimal evidence on which many of these ideas are based and yet which attract huge popular interest. For example, so-called 'miracle cures' such as herbal remedies and fruit drinks are advertised and sold and yet the evidence underpinning their medicinal qualities is often unproven. Goldacre writes especially ardently on the 'science' of detoxification, and outlines the lack of good quality evidence supporting any benefits of this widely used practice. Goldacre gives many examples where 'weighing up' or critical appraisal of the evidence has not been carried out, and, as a result, many people are adhering to practices or beliefs that have no scientific underpinning. In other words, there is very little evidence behind some of these popular 'remedies', and it is important that people think critically and question them, rather than take at face value the claims made by those who profit financially from their use.

An example of critical thinking in action

To be a critical thinker, you need to be able to understand and make sense of what you read, see and hear. As a professional, bombarded with a vast amount of information/evidence, you will come across sources of information that conflict with each other. You need to understand why this is the case in order to make sense of the information. This is a long-term goal and you are not expected to understand all the complex information, literature and evidence you come across right from the outset. However, if you start by developing the right skills, you will become more and more adept at doing this.

In **Example 3**, we consider a statement on critical thinking that has been agreed by experts (Facione 2013) and apply it to a specific situation. Facione describes the characteristics of a critical thinker as being someone who does not accept things at face value:

The ideal critical thinker is habitually inquisitive, well-informed, trustful of reason, open-minded, flexible, fair-minded in evaluation, honest in facing personal biases, prudent in making judgments, willing to reconsider, clear about issues, orderly in complex matters, diligent in seeking relevant information, reasonable in the selection of criteria, focused in inquiry, and persistent in seeking results which are as precise as the subject and the circumstances of inquiry permit.

(2013: 26)

Example 3: Critical thinking in action

In this example, we demonstrate how you can use critical thinking. Imagine that your patient or client has read the following news report in a leading current affairs publication. She asks you for your views on the report:

Kedmey, D. (2014) Do mammograms save lives? 'Hardly', a new study finds, *Time Magazine*, 12 February.

The first thing you might note is the date of the research paper. Whilst papers published some time ago will not necessarily have been replaced by more recent research, it is important to be aware of the possibility of more recent research.

The news item claimed that a study by Miller et al. (2014) had come to the 'startling conclusion' that mammograms 'appear to be useless, at best'. The news item describes a study that compared the outcome for women who had been randomly assigned to receive either a mammogram or a breast examination. The study had found that women who had received just breast examination fared no worse than those who had mammography in the detection of breast cancer. The conclusion made was that mammograms do not save lives.

But is this really the appropriate conclusion to be made about this study? We suggest that by applying a critical approach, you may come to a different conclusion, one that will benefit your patient or client. **Inquisitive and open-minded,** you remember attending a lecture about the benefits of screening, not only for breast cancer but also for many other diseases. This news report seems to question the benefits. Feeling somewhat confused, you endeavour to find out more. You realize you cannot respond to your patient/client's request from the information presented and – demonstrating Facione's requirement of **persistence** – you decide to seek further information/evidence in order to be *well informed.*

The first thing you should do is to consider the quality of the evidence you have been presented with. Don't be tempted to accept the headline that you have been shown as fact. You need further information. Indeed, Facione tells us to be diligent in seeking further information. Remember that a current affairs journal article reporting a study – even if the journal is reputable – may not be an accurate representation of that study. It certainly does not provide sufficient evidence upon which you should inform your patient or client, and so it should trigger further action on your part.

The most useful step to take is to access the original research paper (Miller et al. 2014). We will discuss what research is and how you recognize it in later chapters of this book. For now, let us see how the full report of a systematic scientific investigation or project (which is generally what research is) is likely to be stronger evidence, and will give you more information, than a report in a magazine or journal. You access the original research paper:

ORIGINAL RESEARCH: Miller, A.B., Wall, C., Baines, C.J., Sun, P., To, T. and Narod, S.A. (2014) Twenty five year follow-up for breast cancer incidence and mortality of the Canadian National Breast Screening Study: randomised screening trial, *British Medical Journal,* 348: g366.

To find the research report, you need to search for and locate the article to which the news report is referring using subject-specific search engines (we will discuss how to do this in Chapter 3). This is demonstrating Facione's characteristic of persistence, as you don't easily give up.

When you locate the research, you find that it is a large randomized controlled study in which healthy women had been randomized to receive either a mammogram or physical breast examination on a regular basis. Both groups were followed up over many years and the incidence of

> breast cancer in both groups was measured. The researchers found that those women who had physical examination only, had very similar outcomes to those who had mammography; that is, there was an equal rate of breast cancer-related deaths in the two groups.
>
> You return to the news report in *Time Magazine* and consider the wording. You now feel that 'Does mammography save lives? Hardly' was misrepresentative and possibly sensationalist. A more accurate statement would be that both mammography and physical breast examination seem to save lives.
>
> Such doubt on the value of mammography could perhaps be justified if the researchers had compared mammography with absolutely no intervention and the two groups of women had fared equally (although this would probably have been unethical). But instead, they compared mammography against another method of detecting breast abnormalities. They found that women in both groups fared about the same. Returning to your patient or client, you can now explain that there is evidence from a large study that physical breast examination is as effective at detecting breast cancer as mammography but that there might be other factors to consider – for example, this is a long-term study and the effectiveness of mammograms in detecting breast cancer may have improved over time.

From **Example 3**, you can see why it is so important to be a critical thinker and a critical reader. In working through this example, you can see how, as a critical thinker, you can *make sense of complex issues* (Facione 2013). This enables you to get behind the headlines to see what the evidence is really telling you. You can see how a news report alone is not sufficient evidence upon which to base practice or recommendations to patients or clients. It is important to dig beneath titles and headlines to find out what the information is really about. This example thus illustrates the importance of accessing the best available information/evidence about the situation you are concerned with. We discuss this in Chapters 2 and 3.

How you can think more critically – using our 'Six questions for critical thinking'

We cannot stress enough how important it is to challenge your own assumptions and consider whether you hold any biases that might affect your views or perspectives on a topic. As practice in health and social care has a strong (although not exclusive) evidence-based focus, it is also important to read and ask questions about what people tell you, and also to learn to make sense of what you read, see or hear. We will now introduce our '**Six questions for critical thinking**' to assist you. You will often come across the following key terms:

Critical thinking is when you adopt a questioning approach and thoughtful attitude to what you read, see or hear, rather than accepting things at face value. It also involves challenging your own and others' assumptions. This relates to both academic work and professional practice. 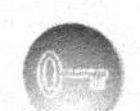

Critical thinking involves a *critical analysis and appraisal* of the information/evidence available to you.

*Critical analysis is when you break down or explore in depth all the components of the information/evidence you have. You can use questions 1–5 of our '**Six questions for critical thinking**' to help you do this. This may involve exploring what is happening and the reasons why. You may need to consider alternative perspectives, including theory, the opinions of others and research findings (see **Examples 1, 2** and **3** earlier in this chapter).* 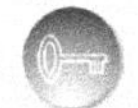

*Critical appraisal is when you consider the strengths and limitations of the information/evidence you read, see and hear, depending on the type of evidence you have. When you start to think critically, you will also begin to critically appraise the information available to you. You can use all of our '**Six questions for critical thinking**' to help you do this, with emphasis on the questions in italics.* 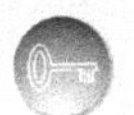

Professional judgement is when you consider, appraise information/evidence and evaluate whether, and to what extent, it is relevant to the care of your patient(s)/client(s). The end result of professional judgement is usually a decision about the optimum care of a patient or client. 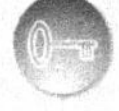

Introducing our 'Six questions for critical thinking'

The following six questions have been adapted from a tool originally devised by Woolliams et al. (2009). We have further adapted and updated this tool based on feedback from staff and students. You can use the six questions to help you consider the type of evidence/information you have and the strengths and weaknesses of any piece of information/evidence you come across (e.g. news items, research reports, discussions with colleagues, and so on). The questions will help you to judge the quality of the information/evidence and therefore help you to decide how or whether to use it in your practice or academic work.

How to use this tool

There is no exact way to assess the relevance of information – this remains for you to judge. But our **'Six questions for critical thinking**' will help you in this process. As a general rule, research studies will provide you with stronger evidence than more anecdotal literature, and information from experts will be stronger than information from people with less experience. Also, recent high-quality literature will be stronger than older literature, but no literature is perfect. We discuss this in more detail in another book in this series, *A Beginner's Guide to Evidence Based Practice in Health and Social Care*, 4th edition (Aveyard et al. 2023).

Some additional notes about our 'Six questions for critical thinking'

What is it? It is very important that you can recognize the type of information/evidence that you have. Wallace and Wray (2016) place information into four categories: research, practice, theory and policy. In general, well-conducted research is the strongest form of evidence and frequently relied on in health and social care. For all types of information/evidence, you need to judge the quality of the arguments or evidence presented. It is also important to be able to summarize the findings.

Where did you find it? Sometimes you might come across a link to an academic paper on social media. Whether you are doing an assignment or dissertation, or searching for evidence to inform practice, it is important to get the best available information/evidence rather than relying on what first comes to hand (see later chapters where we discuss how to search for evidence).

Who has written/said this? It is important to identify whether the authors include their relevant qualifications and have the experience to write or speak authoritatively on the topic. For research, it is also important that they have the necessary clinical, professional and/or academic expertise to undertake the research.

When was it written/said? It is important to consider the date of information/publication. Older information will still be valid if it is considered 'key or seminal' (i.e. it is still widely referenced and used in more recent texts). However, you should determine whether there are newer theories or research that may be equally or more valid.

Why was it written/said? It is important to consider that information will be tailored differently to meet the different needs of different groups. You should also consider any agendas, conflicts or incentives (hidden or open).

How do you know if it is good quality? This question incorporates all of those above in addition to consideration of the overall quality or **analysis** of the information/evidence. Consider whether the arguments presented are robust and, if the information/evidence is research, whether the method is appropriate to the study. Some understanding of research methods is useful here and a research methods textbook will help you develop your understanding. A summary of research methods is given in *A Beginner's Guide to Evidence Based Practice in Health and Social Care*, 4th edition (Aveyard et al. 2023).

Discussing the type of information you refer to in an assignment or report

We suggest that you get used to citing some detail about the information that you use in your academic or professional work (e.g. in an **essay**, report or presentation). For example, if the information you use in an assignment is a research report, say so. If it is anecdotal information or professional opinion, let your reader/audience know this. This lets readers/listeners know that you understand the type of information/evidence you are using. You should use the best source of information/evidence available. We discuss this in Chapter 4.

<table>
<tr><td colspan="2">

Six questions for thinking critically about information/evidence

(**'Six questions for critical thinking'** Version 4, adapted by the authors from Woolliams et al. 2009)

How to use this tool

Use the following **'Six questions'** to help you analyse and appraise verbal or written information/evidence in practice and education.

</td></tr>
<tr><td>

1. **What** is it?
    - What type of evidence is it? For example, is it a literature review, a research study, guidelines, personal opinion, a discussion paper, a website, or another type of evidence?
    - What are the findings/results or key points and are they relevant to what you want to know?

</td><td></td></tr>
<tr><td>

2. **Where** did you find it?
    - Did you just 'come across' it? Who told you? Or did you access it through a systematic search using a professional database?

</td><td></td></tr>
<tr><td>

3. **Who** has written/said this?
    - Are they an individual representing their own viewpoint, or are they an individual/group representing an organization?
    - Are they expert(s) in the topic? How do you know?

</td><td></td></tr>
<tr><td>

4. **When** was this written/said?
    - Older key information may still be valid, but you need to check if there has been more recent work.

</td><td></td></tr>
<tr><td>

5. **Why** has this been written/said?
    - Who is the information aimed at – public, professionals or patient/client groups?
    - What is the aim of the information? Could there be a hidden agenda?
    - Could there be any bias? How do you know?

</td><td></td></tr>
<tr><td>

6. **How** do you know if it is good quality?
    - How were the conclusions reached? Are the research methods used and/or line of reasoning logical, robust and understandable? Are there any flaws in the arguments or approach?

</td><td></td></tr>
<tr><td>

So what?

- **Is this the 'best available' evidence to inform your academic writing and/or practice?**
- **Is this enough information or do you need to find out more?**
- **How will this now impact on your thinking and practice?**

</td><td></td></tr>
</table>

Figure 1.2 Six questions for critical thinking

The need to think critically has never been more important …

There are two reasons for this. First, there has been a marked growth in our **professional knowledge** due to the increase in available evidence and the emphasis on **evidence-based practice**. Second, health and social care professionals are increasingly **accountable** for their practice.

Critical thinking and the increase in professional knowledge

We live in a world in which the pace of change is often so rapid that what is published today may be out of date by the time you read it. This is just as true in health and social care as in any other setting. What you learn today in a lecture or in the workplace might be out of date by the time you encounter a situation in which you put this new knowledge into practice. It is certainly true that change is happening all the time and we would argue that you should embrace change. One reason why there is constant change is that we are continuously acquiring new information/evidence about health and social care topics. Of course, not all of this information/evidence will be good quality, and you need to be discerning about what you use in professional practice in order to make good decisions about patient and client care.

What is evidence-based practice?

You may have heard the term 'evidence-based practice'. Evidence-based practice is about being able to provide a strong **rationale** for your health or social care practice.

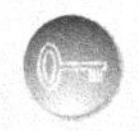

Put simply: 'Evidence based practice is practice that is supported by clear reasoning, taking into account the patient's/client's preferences and using your own judgement' (Aveyard et al. 2023: 4).

The importance of the concept of evidence-based practice is that it emphasizes the need for the best possible evidence to underpin practice. The concept of evidence-based practice has replaced the concept of practice based on tradition and ritual. Most definitions of evidence-based practice argue that in addition to evidence, professionals should use their professional judgement alongside consideration of patient or client preferences (Aveyard et al. 2023).

Information overload and knowledge management

Together with the rise in interest in evidence-based practice, there has been a vast increase in knowledge and other evidence relating to professional practice and discussion about how this should be managed. Some information is useful and some less so. There is so much information available on any health or social care matter that it can be difficult to read and comprehend everything related to your topic of study, let alone work out if the information is of good quality. This is why you need to be a critical thinker – so that you can work out what is useful information and what is less useful for your practice and academic writing.

Example

In an earlier example, we referred to the work of Pertwee et al. (2022), who estimated the number of tweets that were made about the COVID-19 epidemic and the importance of being a critical recipient of information. Information overload is nothing new. Back in 2010, the *British Medical Journal* published a paper by Fraser and Dunstan who cited the example of a cardiac surgeon who would need to read 40 papers each day, every day for 11 years to keep abreast of new developments in their field. Of course, at the end of the 11 years, these developments would already be out of date! Furthermore, as time has gone by and more research has become available, these estimates will have increased, emphasizing the impossibility of keeping up to date with all research in your area.

This situation is roughly the same in every health and social care field. In addition to published academic papers, there are new websites, blogs and information resources for patients/clients. If you do a quick internet search on any health or social care topic using a search engine such as Google, you will get many thousands of results or 'hits'. This will be far too many to make any sense of, and this is why you require a *more specific professional health or social care* **database** (which we discuss in Chapter 3) rather than a general internet search engine when searching more seriously for health or social care topics. Using a more specific database will reduce the number of unwanted hits you get; however, you will still access many thousands of hits unless you are very focused in your search.

Take, for example, the topic of dementia, one that is potentially relevant to health and social care professionals. CINAHL is the abbreviated title of a well-used database containing references for health and social care. We discuss the use of this database in Chapter 3. A general search for information about dementia using this subject-specific database will yield thousands of hits. If you are more specific and request only *research papers* about dementia, you will still get a few thousand hits. Reducing this further to a particular aspect of dementia care will reduce the number of hits still further, but they are still likely to run into many hundreds or a few thousand. Clearly, this is a daunting number, but it illustrates the point we are trying to make – the more focused your search is, the more you can narrow down your search and reduce the number of unwanted hits you get.

Consider one area of your professional or clinical practice (it could be a patient/client problem or intervention) and think of a key phrase related to it. Enter the key phrase into a database or search engine and see how many results (hits) you get. How do you think this would compare with 10 or 20 years ago? 

You can see that if you are going to use evidence in your professional practice and academic writing, you need to seek out the best available information for your studies and practice. You also need to focus on the specific aspect of the topic you are interested in so that you do not get side-tracked with more general information and therefore fail to find out what you really need to know. You also need to be selective about what you read, see and hear and be able to recognize good quality evidence when you come across it. It is also important to make sense of what you read, see and hear, so that you can work out what information is good quality and should influence your practice, and what isn't and should not. In general, research will be stronger evidence than **anecdotal evidence** and **reviews of research** will be stronger still. We will discuss these in more detail in Chapter 3.

Smith (2010) describes the responses from some health and social care workers to managing vast amounts of information. He highlights two main strategies: the 'ostrich strategy' that is adopted by those who do not try to keep up to date, and the 'pigeon strategy' in which professionals 'cherry pick' what they want to believe from all the available information. This 'pigeon' approach might include listening only to what they hear from colleagues in practice and not finding out more from a range of sources. In this book, we argue that neither strategy is appropriate: it is not good practice to accept the first thing you read, see or are told in practice without further investigation. You need to be more critical than this.

Professional knowledge is changing and expanding all the time. It is not possible to teach everyone how to respond in every given clinical and professional situation. As information/evidence is increasing at such a fast pace, all students/learners and practitioners need to be confident in accessing new knowledge, and they need to be able to think critically about it. Professionals need skills to access and interpret the knowledge they require when they require it. We will not survive in professional life if we simply try to remember facts or learn from experience, as we will quickly become out of date. Furthermore, we will then be 'role-modelling' out-of-date practice for others to learn from. It doesn't take much imagination to see how practice can quickly become outdated if people learn from others who are not up to date. We need to keep up to date and respond flexibly and creatively to solve problems in fast-changing health and social care environments.

In response to this information overload, the best strategy is not just to keep reading and accessing up-to-date information but also to *be critical of the information* you read, so that you know which information is useful to you and which is less useful. The aim of this book is to show you how to do this most effectively.

It is not appropriate in the world of health and social care to accept everything you are told by lecturers and practice assessor/mentors, or to learn only by observing role models and building up experience. You also need to:

- **Read widely** about your topic and appraise the quality of what you are reading.
- **Think critically** about what you see and hear in practice.
- **Think critically** about how you seek out and use good quality information from a variety of sources.
- **Think critically** about how the best new evidence can be applied to your practice.

Professional accountability

*Check and see how your organization and/or professional body pro- 
motes accountability and/or critical thinking. If not explicit, consider
further how your practice decisions or interventions are guided by
your own beliefs and/or values and/or by professional policy and
guidelines.*

In many countries around the world, the accountability of health and
social care professionals is an integral part of professional standards
or codes of conduct. As a health or social care professional or student/
learner, you may have a representative professional governing body.
For example, professional bodies in the UK, including the Nursing and
Midwifery Council (NMC 2018) and the Health and Care Professions
Council (HCPC 2012), emphasize the importance of accountability for
professional practice. There is often further guidance in specific professional colleges, associations and organizations, or in job descriptions or
policies provided by your employer.

As a practitioner, you must be able to justify and give a clear account
of and rationale for your practice, and this means that you are answerable for your acts and your omissions. This involves a duty to provide
the most up-to-date care, based on the best available evidence. It is the
role of the professional to incorporate relevant information into everyday practice in order to provide *safe and effective* patient/client care and
to ensure that the best care is delivered. A key component of accountability is thinking critically about your practice and being able to justify
your actions and decisions.

When you are called to account for your practice, you will only be
able to do so if you have administered care that you can justify. It is
no good trying to defend yourself by saying, 'my colleague advised me
to do this' or 'my lecturer told me to do that'. This will not be seen as
a good justification for your actions, and would certainly not be seen
as a strong defence. It is not difficult to see where this is taking us.
There is an ever-increasing amount of information available for health
and social care professionals to make sense of, and each professional
has an obligation to make decisions based on the best available evidence in order to provide optimum care and remain accountable to
their professional body. The best way to defend your practice is
to provide appropriate evidence to justify your actions – you need to
be able to think critically to be able to do this. We discuss this further
in Chapter 5.

> A **common feature** of all professional organizations is that they empha-
> size that those accountable to them should (a) provide a high standard
> of practice at all times, and (b) provide care based on the best avail-
> able evidence. This requires you to **think critically**.

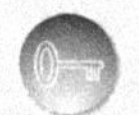

One reason it is important to make sense of the information you come across is that, as a health or social care professional, you are account-able for the care you give. If you are thinking critically about your practice, you are more likely to be able to fully justify the decisions you make and the interventions you carry out.

The complicated part comes when you consider that most aspects of care are informed by a wealth of information: recent developments, experience, expert opinion, research, policy documents, standards of practice, and so on. For any one aspect of care, there is a vast amount of information, including literature to consider. Once you have all the relevant information, you need to be critical of what you read, see and hear, and then make a judgement about it so that you can account for your care or practice if called on to do so.

Who are you accountable to?

- Students are accountable to their higher education institution, and when in a practice setting should be supervised by a registered professional.
- Registered practitioners are usually accountable to their professional body and their employers.
- All registered health and social care practitioners are accountable to the law.

What about your legal responsibilities?

We all have a moral and ethical responsibility to deliver health and social care in a safe and effective way. In many countries, professionals owe a legal duty of care to those they look after and this duty involves delivering care that is based on the best available evidence.

In many countries, recent case law has supported the role of evidence, and using the best available evidence, to determine the standard of care that professionals have to deliver rather than allowing professionals to disregard evidence and set their own standards. Overturning a previous landmark case (*Bolam* v. *Friern Hospital Management Committee* [1957] 2 All ER 118 per McNair J.), judges have ruled that a doctor has a duty to use the best available evidence rather than rely on an outdated defence of 'this is what my colleagues do'. In the case of *Bolitho* v. *City & Hackney Health Authority* [1993] 13 BMLR 111, CA, the court held that the body of expert opinion relied upon to judge good practice should be logical and evidence-based, thus establishing a legal duty to provide care that is based on the best available evidence, rather than a repetition of other professionals' action or advice.

See if you can find any examples of legal cases where a health or social care professional has been prosecuted or litigated against. Consider whether a lack of critical thinking may have contributed to the reasons why the case arose.

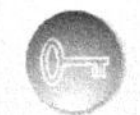

If you think critically about your practice and critically appraise evidence, you will be equipped to practise in a safe and effective way. You will also be more likely to be able to justify and account for your decisions and interventions.

How critical thinking can help you in your professional practice and academic assignments

We have illustrated how we are often inundated with information, but a lot of it is of poor quality and we therefore need to think critically about the information we are presented with. **Examples 1** and **2** earlier in the chapter also helped illustrate how it is easy for a critical approach to be lost within a 'good story'. While this is unfortunate within everyday life, it is far worse and potentially far more serious within health and social care practice, as professionals risk making poor decisions if they are not critical about the information upon which they base their practice. Critical thinking is a skill that is essential to acquire and one that will enhance your practice. We illustrated this in **Example 3**.

As a student or professional undertaking further education, if you examine the marking criteria for your academic assignments, you will see that you are marked on your ability to demonstrate that you can be critical of the literature you include. This involves using the best available evidence relating to the points you are making and writing with a critical voice. In principle, this generally means looking for research evidence rather than anecdotal sources. We also have to be aware of what constitutes good quality research and if, at all possible, look for reviews of research rather than individual papers. This is because a review of research provides a summary of all the papers on a topic: one individual piece of research is just one piece of the jigsaw. It is also necessary to make a judgement about the quality of the sources you use, which we will explain in later chapters. In your professional practice, this means questioning what you are told and looking up information to inform the care you give. Taking information at face value and out of context – even if it is stated by an expert colleague or published in a reputable professional journal – is not the way to attain academic or professional credibility.

The need for health and social care professionals to keep up to date with information about new developments, and appraise the merits of new research and proposals in relation to their own practice, is one of the main drivers behind the current move in the UK and other countries towards an 'all-graduate' health and social care professional body. The need to be able to think critically as a safe, effective and independent practitioner has never been greater. Qualified professionals will be individuals who are able to assess the patient/client, plan and evaluate evidence-based care which can then be implemented by others, including assistant practitioners, care assistants and those in supportive roles. As professionals, we need to be critical thinkers in order to plan and evaluate the effectiveness of the interventions we deliver rather than carrying out care unquestioningly.

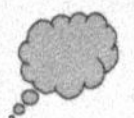

Before you move on to the rest of the book, can you identify how you might become more critical in your practice or academic writing?

Because there is so much information available, in this book we make a distinction between information that is readily available (e.g. lecture notes, recommended textbooks or the opinion of colleagues – which we discuss in Chapter 2) and information for which you need to search a bit harder, such as through a literature search to locate relevant research studies and reviews (which we discuss in Chapter 3).

It is important to note that we will be discussing critical thinking in relation to both your professional practice *and* academic studies.

We will also discuss some steps to take to become a critical academic writer. This is because practice and theory are closely interconnected. Sometimes you may be writing about what you or others have done in your workplace, or you may be applying knowledge or research gained from writing in relation to your management of care for a patient/client. It is hoped that this book will assist you in developing your skills as a critical thinker within health and social care. Read on …

In summary

Being a critical thinker helps us to make rational decisions. We need to examine our own beliefs, such as our preconceived ideas, assumptions, values and biases, in order to think critically about the information we come across. There is a vast amount of information and evidence that you will encounter, and you will need to make sense of what you see, hear and read and not accept arguments at face value. We have suggested an approach to being critical using our '**Six questions for critical thinking**'. As a professional, you are accountable and you should ensure that the practice you deliver is evidence-based. Critical thinking helps us to work out which evidence to use.

Key points

1   Critical thinking is essential to promote the best decision-making.
2   Critical thinking means being critical about the information we receive and how we use it.
3   Information is expanding in all areas of health and social care – some information is useful and relevant, some less so, and some can be inaccurate or misleading.
4   As professionals we need to be able to work out which information is useful to us and use it appropriately.
5   We suggest using the '**Six questions for critical thinking**' tool. This should help you to identify the most appropriate sources and enable you to be more critical of the information you use in your academic work and professional practice.

2 Thinking more critically about readily available information

- *Critical thinking and the use of information/evidence*
- *What types of information are readily available?*
- *Thinking critically about the quality and usefulness of 'readily available' information*
- *In summary*
- *Key points*

In this chapter, we will:

- Identify what is readily available information.
- Discuss how to judge the quality and usefulness of this information.
- Show how you can begin to think critically about the information you find and how to use it.

Critical thinking and the use of information/evidence

If critical thinking involves challenging your own assumptions and then adopting a questioning approach and thoughtful attitude to what you read, see or hear, then clearly the information/evidence you use in your professional life is very important. As evidence-based practice is a corner-stone of contemporary health and social care practice, we emphasize how you can be critical of evidence throughout this book. We distinguish between information/evidence that is readily available and the best available infor-mation/evidence, which you might have to search a little bit harder for.

What types of information are readily available?

In this chapter, we will look at the information that you will encounter on a day-to-day basis and we will refer to this as **readily available infor-mation**. By this we mean information that you do not have to search long and hard for; you may just encounter it in your day-to-day profes-sional or student life. We all use this type of information/evidence all the time, and it is important to be critical of what you come across. Because there is so much of this information, it is important you can make sense of it and determine whether it is of a good enough quality for you to base your professional practice on or use in your academic work, and when you need to dig a bit deeper.

Think quickly and jot down all the places/people from which you cur-rently get your information related to your studies and/or your practice. 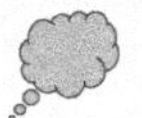

Such forms of 'readily available' information include:

* Social media such as TikTok, Instagram, Threads, X (formerly Twitter).
* Newspapers and other forms of media.
* Internet search engines such as Google and Bing.
* Websites focusing on health and social care.
* Advice from lecturers or practice assessor/mentors.
* Lectures and lecture notes.
* Textbooks.
* Journals to which you have access.
* Professional policies and guidelines.
* Information leaflets by patient or client organizations.

It is important to note that wherever you live in the world, patients/cli-ents may also be exposed to such 'readily available' information and they often use the internet for additional sources of information and a second opinion about their health or social care issues. There are some well-advertised and readily available sources where the public can seek information, including leaflets produced by professional organizations and via the internet – for example, in the UK:

- The British Broadcasting Corporation (BBC) for health news [http://www.bbc.co.uk/news/health/]
- Citizens Advice for a wider range of issues [http://www.citizensadvice.org.uk/]
- Organizations that are targeted at the public include Patient.co.uk [http://www.patient.co.uk/], Patient Opinion [https://www.patientopinion.org.uk/] and NHS Choices [http://www.nhs.uk/Pages/HomePage.aspx].

The problem with 'readily available' information is that there is so much of it! This is partly the result of the information revolution and the free publication of ideas on the internet. Anyone can publish anything online, and you need to be a critical reader to determine whether what you are reading is a reliable source of information. For example, anyone can add or edit information on Wikipedia [http://en.wikipedia.org/wiki/Main_Page], so you cannot be sure whether information about health and social care issues has been submitted by a reliable or knowledgeable source.

Thinking critically about the quality and usefulness of 'readily available' information

Let us look at some sources of 'readily available' information to determine whether they are reliable enough for you to use in your professional practice and academic writing. Remember to use the '**Six questions for critical thinking**' to work out the strengths and weaknesses of the information at your disposal.

Newspapers/news websites

In Chapter 1, we provide an example of how newspapers can use misleading statistics to promote a story. This should be enough of a warning against using media information in your academic work or any practice situation without seeking further information. However, newspapers may provide useful background information. For example, they might lead you to a controversial quotation to start your assignment or to get you thinking more widely. Or they might refer you to a research study, giving a snippet of information but not the full reference for the study, making it harder (but possible) to track it down. In principle, you should avoid direct reference to newspaper articles in your written work or discussions at work unless you use them as a springboard for further enquiry, or you are discussing the media's view or perspective on a topic. Some newspapers may have stricter editorial quality control than others and so may offer a higher standard of information, but it will still need to be checked out. Take, for example, *The Guardian*'s article on 'Hard to swallow: the world's first drinkable sunscreen' (Burnett 2014) – this would certainly warrant further scrutiny.

Internet sources and general search engines

The internet is a fantastic tool that can be used to search for both 'easy to access' and 'harder to find' sources of information/evidence (the latter we discuss in Chapter 3); you can use it to access professional databases, full-text research studies, policies and guidelines, social media, news stories and more general websites. Often a general search engine (such as Google) is the first port of call for busy professionals; however, such a search will not necessarily be able to access good quality evidence. Furthermore, the information presented in the results list from a general search does not prioritize the information for your purposes or order the information in terms of quality, credibility or even relevance. So, unless you use an appropriate **search strategy** and professional database, as discussed in Chapter 3, you are unlikely to get the best and most relevant research from a random internet search. Sometimes you can use general search engines if you know what professional source you are looking for – a reference to a journal article that may be available online, for example. A critical thinker will access the best information in a systematic and professional way.

Websites

The internet provides access to a vast array of websites offering millions of pages of information, including everything from rigorous research to trivia, personal opinion and misinformation. Useful websites are likely to be those that are produced by recognized organizations, professional or patient/client groups. These might contain policies, guidelines for practice, up-to-date news on professional issues, and issues of concern to patient and client groups. But, as with all websites, it is important to recognize quality and possible bias; that is, the presentation of information from a particular viewpoint which is not independently verified.

How can you think critically about the quality of a website?

Before making use of information found on the web in your academic work or practice, you need to make sure it is of a high quality and up to date. Remember to use the '**Six questions for critical thinking**' given in Chapter 1. For example:

What is the evidence that is reported? If a website refers to the conclusion of a piece of research, you should try and access the *original* research if you are using this in your assignments or practice.

Who has authored the website? Note if any author's name is given. If so, consider whether the author is a credible expert on the topic and if they are likely to be biased or have a 'hidden agenda' on the topic – for example, are they from a campaign group trying to get a particular drug or vaccination banned (consider the publicity surrounding the MMR vaccination mentioned in Chapter 1). Is the author's perspective their personal perspective?

When was the site produced? Do not assume it is up to date just because it is still on the internet. See if you can locate the date it first appeared.

Who is the target audience? Remember to use the information in this context. It may be pitched for patients/clients rather than for professionals.

In general, before you use a website in your academic work, you must assess the quality of the site and whenever possible you should use original sources. Consider whether it is the best evidence available or whether you should use it as a springboard for finding further information/ evidence. Citing websites without judging their quality is like telling the marker, 'I was in a bit of a rush and this is all I could find …', and your mark will undoubtedly reflect this. Similarly, if you go to your professional practice area with only a website as a recommendation for change, you will probably be encouraged to find stronger evidence. Remember that if you use information from the web, the relevant web page(s) must be cited in full in your reference list. You may wish to check whether your organization or university has a guide to referencing web pages.

Social media

Social media is being used increasingly in a professional or academic capacity and also by patients. The value of social media is that it is generally accessible to everyone and has enormous potential for sharing ideas and making connections. However, it is a powerful tool and you do need to consider who the influencers are and whether the information provided is balanced (Elson et al. 2021). Our **six questions** to trigger critical thinking can be useful here. You should therefore think critically about how you use social media in your professional capacity, especially if you use it to access sources of information. Common sites used are X (formerly Twitter) [www.X.com (formerly Twitter.com), Facebook [https://www.facebook.com] and, for career networking, LinkedIn [https://www.linkedin.com/]. Many other sites are also available.

Twitter/X enables people to discuss professional issues and even organize professional discussions. It can be used as a learning tool, to converse and share ideas. In addition, it can be used as a source of data – X (formerly Twitter) accounts have been analysed for trends regarding suicide ideology and attitudes to blood donation (Luo et al. 2020; Ramondt et al. 2020). An X (formerly Twitter) user has a username beginning with the '@' symbol. Each contribution or 'tweet' must be a pre-defined set of characters. There are international organizations who use X (formerly Twitter) to communicate important health and policy information; (e.g. @WHO), professional journals tweet about their latest papers, and professional organizations also use X (formerly Twitter) and other social media sites to share information quickly and concisely. You can search on X (formerly Twitter) for topics or people, and you can use hashtags to locate particular discussions (e.g. #critical thinking, #evidence-based practice). Patients or clients may tweet about their experiences of health and social care; for example, under the username @patientopinion you may find patients/carers tweeting about individual topics, and you can search X (formerly Twitter) for a specific topic using a hashtag.

A site that organizes weekly and fortnightly X (formerly Twitter) chats is http://www.wenurses.com/about/index.php. There are specific groups for mental health, midwives, pharmacists, paramedics, learning disability nurses, school nurses and commissioners. There is also information on taking part in X (formerly Twitter) chats.

Blogs (or web logs) are an internet-based forum for people who have opinions or expertise in a particular area. They use blogs to express their ideas – in more words than X (formerly Twitter) – or to draw attention to their own or others' publications and ideas, and increasingly so in education and research. Blogs and tweets are easily disseminated – often via X (formerly Twitter), or you can find them by using a search engine. Many people take to social media to draw attention to issues that they feel strongly about; for example, the 'Hello My Name Is' campaign, initiated by the late Dr Kate Granger, which encouraged all health and care professionals to introduce themselves to their patients using their first name. Blogs and X (formerly Twitter) may offer very different perspectives, specifically on rapidly changing situations or issues.

Importance of critical thinking when using social media

As with any other source, you should think critically about any information/evidence you find on social media. Opinions can be stated very rapidly without users taking time to think through their point or explaining themselves clearly. Thus it is hard to identify which comments on social media are based on consideration of the best available evidence. There are reports in the media of professionals who have been disciplined for unprofessional content on social media sites (Keogh 2013). Levati (2014) found that many nurses' use of social media highlighted a blurring of personal and professional lives, although there are guidelines and warnings against doing this. In the UK, the Nursing and Midwifery Council (NMC 2023a) and the Health and Care Professions Council (HCPC 2024) have guidelines on professional use of social media. Social media may be most useful for individual or personal perspectives and you should recognize it as such. It is important to take into account the context in which it is written. The example of the use of social media to express misinformation about the COVID-19 epidemic, as discussed in Chapter 1, is a clear example of this.

Advice from practice assessors/mentors and colleagues

Practice assessors/mentors and colleagues are a good source of professional knowledge and skills through role modelling. A role model may be described as someone who is able to exemplify behaviour and social roles (Perry 2009). Felstead (2013) notes that practice staff also model professional behaviour. We can all learn from role modelling from other professionals and most of us can remember a good role model. Indeed, learning from other professionals is a major part of professional education. However, remember that health and social care providers are a wide and diverse group. There are expert practitioners and there are novice practitioners. Some practitioners are thoughtful and reflective about their practice, while others are not. The quality of advice you receive in practice may vary!

How can you 'think critically' about information obtained from social media, practice assessors/mentors or colleagues?

If you read something about an intervention or care decision on social media or are informed by a practice assessor/mentor or colleague, consider the '**Six questions for critical thinking**'. For example, consider whether they are quoting from their own experience or from research evidence or guidelines. Where there is no research evidence relating to a complex and unusual problem, experience and reflective judgement can be very valuable. But you need to decide if it is the best available evidence, and you should endeavour to check its accuracy.

Discussion between professionals about information or research that has been critically appraised is likely to be beneficial. However, it is not always the case that information will be critically appraised by practitioners. Referring back to our discussion of the need to be critical of what you read, see and hear, you need to question what you are told in practice rather than accepting what your practice assessor/mentor or colleague tells or shows you. The examples of the reporting of the COVID-19 story **(Example 1**, Chapter 1) and the MMR vaccination story **(Example 2**, Chapter 1) show how misinformation can easily spread when information is not critically appraised. If you stop to think about this, the implications are enormous. If information or advice is not critically appraised or is based on unfounded rumour, and is then passed unchallenged from one professional to another, that is not demonstrating evidence-based practice and is certainly not applying critical thinking! So beware of accepting information at face value from your practice assessor/mentor and your colleagues. We will discuss this further in Chapter 5.

Lectures or conference presentations

Lectures or conference presentations may only provide a basic introduction or focus on a specific aspect of a topic. To gain a fuller understanding, you are expected to access the given references or reading list and read more broadly around the subject. It cannot be stressed enough how important it is do this. This is necessary even when an expert delivers the conference presentation, since he or she is only presenting a snapshot of their research or ideas.

If you only refer to lecture notes in your assignment or use them as evidence for your practice, it implies that you have not been thinking critically or in depth about the subject. It gives the same message as described previously: 'I was in a rush and did not have time to find evidence related to the lecture'. You would therefore be unlikely to gain high marks in assignments or be able to offer an adequate explanation for your practice decisions. There is one exception to this, which is when a leading authority or expert delivers a lecture/presentation and he or she is delivering material that is yet to be published. Then, and only then, may you quote from this lecture in your assignment or discuss their ideas in practice without finding further supporting information. However, even then, your argument will be stronger if you find related evidence to back up what you write. Although conference presentations can inform you of expert and up-to-date information/evidence, you should try to read more widely around the topics presented.

How can you think critically about the quality of a lecture/presentation?

When you are in a lecture/presentation, consider the '**Six questions for critical thinking**'. Consider the sources that the lecturer is referring to and whether the arguments they present make sense. Our advice is that you should avoid referring only to a lecture/presentation in your written work or practice. Instead, use the ideas presented there and read more widely on some of the references and refer to these. It is far better still to search more widely on the topic, as we will discuss in Chapter 3 – a lecture/presentation should be used as a basis for further reading and investigation.

Unfortunately, a lot of people rely on information they have received in a lecture without doing the appropriate reading. They also rely on this information for years to come. The implications of this are similar to what happens if practice information is passed from one colleague to another without critical thinking. We quickly become out of date. If we are to become independent critical thinkers, we need to move on from this approach and use lectures as they are meant to be used – as launchpads for further reading and discussion.

Textbooks/e-books

Textbooks, especially at undergraduate level, generally provide a springboard for further study. Some textbooks provide a basic overview of current knowledge on a particular area, especially if you are new to a topic. They may provide sound factual information on topics such as anatomy and physiology. Others provide ideas, theoretical models and frameworks or opinions on a topic by leading experts. The main thing is to ensure that you have identified the most appropriate textbook for your purpose.

How do you know if a textbook is a useful one?

We suggest you do not start with a specialist book if you are new to a topic. This is because when you are new to a topic, it is usually most helpful to have an overview of that topic rather than to start by focusing on a specialist area that you may not be able to put into context. Using the '**Six questions for critical thinking**':

- Consider who the author is, the date of publication and the target audience.
- Be prepared to use the textbook as a springboard for further reading.
- Use the information on the back cover to find out who the book is aimed at and what the contents cover.
- Consider whether the textbook is appropriate for your level and focus of study.

We also suggest that you read reviews of textbooks and follow recommendations on your reading list for core texts, noting who these are aimed at. Remember, it may be many months or even years before a book is published, so consider how up to date the information is and whether there are likely to be changes in the evidence used to support the arguments presented there. Finally, make sure that you have the most up-to-date edition of any textbook you use, remembering that new editions of the most popular texts are generally published every few years. Look at the dates of the references cited in the book too. Those who mark your work will notice if you are referring to an older version of a recently updated book.

Hard copy and electronic journals

Research and other information that is published in academic journals forms the basis of much of our professional knowledge, something we discuss in depth in Chapter 3. However, in this chapter, we are interested in 'readily available' sources, and thus information in journals you are not specifically searching for but come across by chance in your everyday life. Many workplaces subscribe to a journal, either in print format or using an online electronic journals facility. If you find this is the case in your work or practice area, find out why that particular journal was chosen. It may be a specialist journal that publishes all the best research in a particular study area. But remember, different information will be available in different journals and thus you might not get the 'whole picture' if you refer to one journal alone. There are also an increasing number of **open access journals** for which you do not need to subscribe, which you may come across from initial internet searches. You should make sure that they have been **peer reviewed** before publication. Peer review is the process by which experts in a subject area are invited to review the academic work of an author, often prior to publication in a journal. Refer to Chapter 3 where we discuss how to search for a wider range of literature.

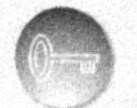

One research paper, even if it is a piece of good quality research relevant to your topic, will rarely be enough for you to base a judgement on regarding correct practice or an academic argument. For any one study supporting a view, there may be four other papers that have a contradictory view.

How can you think critically about what you find in a journal?

A wide variety of information is presented in journals, including editorials, original research papers and letters to the editor. It is important that you can recognize the types of information you come across and use this appropriately in your written work or practice environment. When you apply the '**Six questions for critical thinking**', consider carefully the 'what' so that you are clear about the type of information you have – for example, is it an editorial, a research study (if so, what type?), a descriptive literature review or a systematic review, an overview of the topic? These are explained below. One important thing to remember is that journals that are easily available in your workplace will not provide a comprehensive range of relevant information on a topic. A full range of relevant information may be published in a variety of other sources and you will only find these through carrying out a comprehensive search, which we discuss in Chapter 3.

What information will you find in a journal?

Editorials

Editorials are generally written by the editor of a journal and represent their viewpoint or the viewpoint of the editorial team.

Systematic reviews

These are reviews of published research undertaken on a particular topic and are generally presented using a research structure as presented below. The structure ensures that the method is transparent and repeatable.

- A question or statement of aims
- Method: this should outline the approach to the search and be comprehensive
- Results or findings
- Discussion
- Conclusions.

A systematic review should discuss how the quality of the research was appraised. The most comprehensive collection of systematic reviews is the Cochrane Collaboration and its sister organization, the Campbell

Collaboration. These are reviews compiled by expert 'systematic reviewers' and published on the Cochrane Collaboration website [https://www.cochrane.org], and for more public health-focused information, the Campbell Collaboration website [https://www.campbellcollaboration.org]. Cochrane and Campbell Collaboration reviews usually publish studies exploring 'does it work?' questions and therefore incorporate randomized controlled trials. Do note that the term 'systematic review' is not reserved for this specific type of review; there are other reviews, which have been undertaken systematically, which might be of qualitative or mixed methods studies. The key factor in identifying a systematic review is whether the review has been done in a systematic manner.

Unsystematic reviews or descriptive reviews

These may give a broad overview of a topic, drawing on a wide range of literature. However, unless the approach to finding the literature is thorough and there is a specific question and method for the search, you cannot be sure that all the evidence on the topic has been included and there may be some bias in the selection of studies used; that is, the information included might not have been identified in a systematic way. You should also note whether the quality of the research used has been appraised. This type of review will provide weaker evidence than one that has been compiled systematically. However, that is not to say that the information will not be useful, as such reviews may provide a concise (but not comprehensive) introduction to, or overview of, a topic. If you refer to this type of review in your written work, make sure that you are clear about the type of evidence you are using. You may then want to access the individual research studies or papers referred to in the review.

Research studies

Research studies generally provide stronger evidence than more anecdotal sources. These can easily be identified, as they normally begin with a specific research question (or aim) that is addressed using an identified method, following which the results or findings, discussion and conclusions are presented. Such studies can be quantitative (measuring or counting something) or qualitative (describing something), and various approaches can be adopted with either type of research.

Research studies can provide good sources of evidence but they still need to be appraised individually. Be wary of a single piece of research evidence that makes a claim about practice. Consider a jigsaw where you only have one bit of the picture; sometimes you cannot tell what the final view will be. Instead, as we will discuss in Chapter 3 it is better to search more broadly for further research papers or to locate a systematic review that has already been carried out. This is so that you can gain an overview of what the conclusion should be based on all the research on the topic – that is, complete the whole jigsaw.

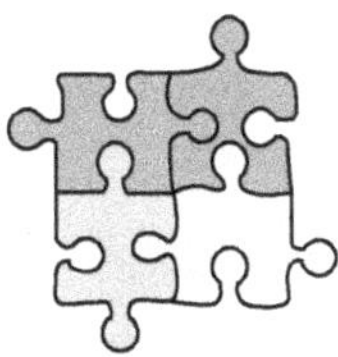

Figure 2.1

Discussion or opinion papers

These will not have as clear a structure as a research study and will be introduced as representing the opinion of the author. Remember that the quality of this type of evidence will depend on the expertise of the person writing the paper – do not assume that even an expert will be basing their argument on relevant and evidence-based sources. Experts might also be biased – not necessarily intentionally – in the selection of the sources they use. Our advice is that you should only use this type of evidence when you cannot find research evidence on your topic or as a starting point for searching for your investigations.

Professional and clinical guidance, policies and 'evidence-based' knowledge summaries

The move towards providing summaries of evidence is one of the most useful developments in health and social care. You might see paper volumes or links to internet sites that summarize the best available evidence.

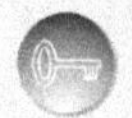

If you come across up-to-date policy or guidelines based on the evidence from systematic reviews or summaries of systematic reviews, you have strong evidence upon which to base your professional practice or academic work.

The above publications are different from other types of 'readily accessible' information because they are based not only on research but also on systematic reviews of research of best available evidence. Below is an example of one of these summaries:

- **Evidence in Health and Social Care** launched in 2009. This has a search facility and ranks research according to relevance and quality [see www.evidence.nhs.uk].

How do you think critically about guidelines or knowledge summaries?

We argue that these kind of guidelines or summaries of best available evidence are an extremely useful resource for your academic and professional practice and they are readily available, usually in the practice environment. So how can you tell which of these guidelines and summaries are of good quality? You can apply the '**Six questions for critical thinking**' to guidelines that you use. Tools have also been developed for the evaluation of guidelines, such as the AGREE 11 tool [available at: http://www.agreetrust.org/], and a tool called DISCERN, which is used to ascertain the quality of written information on treatment choices [see www.discern.org.uk].

Generally, there should be a good explanation of how the guidelines or summaries were compiled. The sources that were used should be clearly identified; these should be from best available evidence, usually research and systematic reviews of research. You should also check if they are up to date and have a review date.

If you come across guidelines and policies that appear to be evidence-based, then these are likely to be strong evidence. This is because guidelines and policies from reliable sources (as in the examples given above) are compiled from the evidence from systematic reviews.

In other words, they have done the hard work of searching for the best available evidence (as we discuss in Chapter 3).

Access the AGREE or DISCERN website and see if you can find some guidelines that are relevant to you in your professional role. 

Remember ...
You should 'think critically' about every source of information that you consider using. 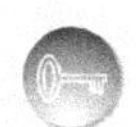

In summary

In this chapter, we have outlined how you need to think critically about the readily available information that you may come across in your everyday life as a student/learner or as a professional. The range of readily available information is vast and it is important that you can judge the quality and relevance of what you find. We have argued that newspaper articles and news items as well as many websites can be misleading and that they should be referred to minimally. They should certainly not be used in the main body of your assignment or as the focus of decision-making within professional practice. Information from practice assessors/colleagues and from lecture notes and social media should be used only as a springboard for further study, rather than as an end in itself. Textbooks and academic journals that you encounter 'at random' may or may not be the most appropriate for your academic and professional learning needs, so consider their use carefully. If you come across a useful article in a journal in your placement area, you need to consider what type of paper it is and whether there are other relevant articles that would add to or help 'complete the picture'. If you find well-developed and well-established guidelines – especially those produced nationally by recognized organizations – you will have some high-quality evidence.

Remember that 'readily available' information is usually just the 'tip of the iceberg' of the total information available on a particular topic. To paint a more comprehensive picture, you need to search more thoroughly, as we will discuss in Chapter 3.

Key points

1   There is a vast amount of 'readily available' information. Such *readily available* evidence generally represents the 'tip of the iceberg' of information available. You need to think critically about this in order to make decisions about the care and support provided to patients and clients based on the best available evidence.
2   This *readily available* information ranges from information that can be inaccurate and misleading to useful sources.
3   Try to avoid referencing media sources or unevaluated websites in your assignments.
4   Use lecture notes and advice from practice assessors/mentors and colleagues as a springboard for further study.
5   Remember that books and articles found in journals need to be viewed alongside other relevant publications.
6   Professional guidelines and summaries of evidence generally provide strong evidence if they are up to date and based on best available evidence.

3 Being more critical: finding the 'best available' evidence

- *Why you need to dig deeper to find evidence*
- *Beginning the search process*
- *Using subject-specific electronic databases*
- *How you can plan and search for literature using specific databases*
- *What is the 'best available' evidence?*
- *Research evidence*
- *In summary*
- *Key points*

In this chapter, we will:

- Explain why you need to dig a little deeper to find the 'best available' evidence in order to promote critical thinking.
- Explore the value of using specific databases to search for evidence, and examine how to plan and search for evidence using specific databases.

- Discuss how to find the best available evidence.
- Discuss what type of research and other information/evidence you should look for and how you will know when you have found it.

Why you need to dig deeper to find evidence

You can see from the discussion in Chapter 2 that you need to think carefully about information that is 'readily available', make a judgement about its quality and decide if you need to dig a little deeper to find the best available evidence. It is then important to think critically and to question the information you find, so that you can recognize the best available evidence when you come across it.

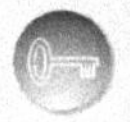

You need to try to ensure you get the whole picture rather than relying on just the first piece of 'readily available' information you find.

We argued in Chapter 2 that unless you come across up-to-date guidelines or policies relating to your practice that are based on the best available evidence, the information that is readily available (that is, information that you do not need to search too hard for) will generally provide just the 'tip of the iceberg' of available information on a topic and is generally best used as a springboard for further investigation or study.

You need to dig deeper because:

- As a 'critical thinker', you should not rely on the most readily available information or opinion; instead, you need to adopt a questioning approach and search for all the available information. Otherwise, you could be making decisions about patients/clients based on weak evidence.
- A piece of research on its own is generally not enough – other studies may provide a different view or, when viewed together, may lead you to a different overall conclusion.
- The quality of information on websites, in the media, on social media and from colleagues may vary and may be biased.
- You need to be certain that you have found all the most up-to-date sources of evidence.
- You should review all the evidence on your topic rather than just select evidence that is in line with your argument.
- More up-to-date and more relevant evidence may recently have become available.

In other words, a systematic and thorough search of relevant health or social care databases will ensure that you have obtained all or most of the evidence on a topic. You will be able to access these databases in your university or hospital library, and we discuss these in this chapter. Undertaking a thorough search for relevant evidence will enable you to demonstrate to the marker of your assignment, or your colleagues in practice, that you have searched diligently for evidence rather than simply relied on readily available sources.

Beginning the search process

In most cases, the best way to search is through your academic or professional library, either online via your library's electronic resources or in person. Without doing this, you are unlikely to access the best available evidence on your topic. Even if you find relevant articles by looking at a recent edition of a journal, you will only be accessing a tiny proportion of evidence that is available on that particular topic. You will not have accessed information that has been published previously or since. You need to ensure that you do not just 'cherry pick' evidence you want to include. You will be demonstrating a *critical approach* when you decide to search more thoroughly for further evidence. This is because you recognize that the evidence you have obtained via readily accessible sources is likely to be insufficient for your purposes.

Why not use Google or other search engines?

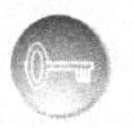

*Internet search engines such as Google are **not** specific enough to search effectively for evidence. Beware of using only sources retrieved through general search engines. Their ability to search is limited and so the information you find may be too broad, of poor quality, or you may have missed a key piece of research.*

Most people are familiar with general internet search engines such as Google. We use them on an everyday basis to search for a wide variety of things. However, they are not specific enough to find the best available professional evidence because they do not distinguish between what is good evidence and what is not. They simply present you with a list of hits and because there is so much information available to you, it is very difficult, if not impossible, to identify what is worth looking at in more depth.

For this reason, for your academic and professional searches you need a search engine that is subject-specific and does not trawl through all the 'lay' publications and other sources of information that relate to your topic. Having said that, doing a quick search using an internet search engine such as Google on a topic you wish to explore further might give you some idea of the terms or language used around your topic. So it might be worth a 'quick look' just to see what words you can then use to search using the more specific professional databases. A slightly more focused search can be carried out on Google Scholar (selected from the 'more' drop-down menu, where you can select type of publication and dates). However, Google Scholar, despite what its name might suggest, does not have access to a full range of academic journals and this will restrict the usefulness of its findings. Hence this would still not constitute a comprehensive search.

Go to a general search engine and search for a health or social care condition or problem and look at the first few results. Then look at results much later in the list. Can you see any difference in the information? Think critically about what the implications would be if you had taken the information/evidence just from the first results.

This indicates how general search engines only provide you with non-specific information/evidence of variable quality.

Using subject-specific electronic databases

To take a critical approach to your academic writing and professional practice, you need to be comprehensive and organized in your search for appropriate evidence. The best way to do this is by using a **subject-specific database**.

> **Why use a subject-specific database instead of a more casual approach to finding literature?**
> - You will find a broader range of literature relevant to your topic – **breadth**.
> - You are more likely to find appropriate literature – **relevance**.
> - You are more likely to find literature of good quality – **rigour**.
> - Your search will be more comprehensive – **thoroughness**.

What is a subject-specific database?

Subject-specific databases hold the references for, and often abstracts or the full text version of, journal articles and many other texts, for which you can search using key words. Many subject-specific databases are related to a particular academic field or professional group(s), such as health and/or social care. They are usually best accessed through your academic or professional library website. A database is simply a way of storing, organizing, searching and accessing information. It is a bit like a large electronic filing cabinet.

Commonly held databases

AMED: Allied health care including complementary medicine

ASSIA: Applied Social Sciences Indexes and Abstracts

Autism Data: Published research papers, books, articles and videos on autism

British Nursing Database: Nursing, midwifery and community health care

Campbell Collaboration: Systematic reviews of the effects of social interventions

CINAHL: Nursing and allied health care from North America and Europe

CIRRIE: Centre for International Rehabilitation Research Information

Cochrane Library: Systematic reviews of evidence-based health care

DARE: Database of Abstracts of Reviews of Effects

HMIC: Non-clinical topics including inequalities in health and user involvement

Joanna Briggs Institute: Nursing-focused systematic reviews

MEDLINE: Extensive medical and nursing database

NICE Clinical Knowledge Summaries: Evidence-based information on common conditions managed in primary care

OpenGREY: Database of grey literature

OTseeker: Abstracts of systematic reviews and RCTs relevant to occupational therapy

Patient experience database: UK collection of evidence on patient experience from a variety of sources

PEDRO: Physiotherapy evidence database

PsycINFO: Psychology, psychiatry, child development and psychological care

PubMed: Medical and health professions

Rehabdata: Disability and rehabilitation

Social Care Online: Social and community care

Social Services Abstracts: Abstracts from journal articles on social work, welfare and policy

Sociological Abstracts: Sociology and political theory

Source: Management and practice of primary health care and disability in developing countries

TRIP database: Evidence-based medicine and health care resources on the web

Web of Science: Includes Science Citation Index and Social Sciences Citation Index

ZETOC: The British Library's electronic table of contents

How to find a subject-specific database

If you go to the website of your academic or professional library, or contact your subject librarian, you are likely to find a list of databases relevant to your field of professional practice. Each database will have a description of its scope and focus – some are psychology related, some are social science based, some are medically focused, while others focus on literature for allied health care professionals, and so on. This is where you need to think creatively and critically in terms of deciding what your focus will be. For example, you need to consider whether information from other professions may add insight and whether you have considered a holistic approach to your issue (e.g. you could consider psychological, cultural or educational issues that may require using a different database). If you are not sure which database to access, ask someone at your local university or from your professional development team.

You could use more than one database if you are doing a very thorough search. If you are not confident using computers, you may find it easier to visit the library in person and access training courses on how to search using databases. Do remember that these databases change their format or their name on a fairly regular basis. If you are resuming a search after a break, check with your subject librarian which database is best for your needs. Also, remember that different databases operate slightly differently, so consult the information provided with the database to ensure that you make full use of the search facility.

Key words and phrases

When you access a database, you will be invited to enter a key word such as 'Dementia' or 'Assessment'. You will then be asked to refine your search using that key word: by date, type of evidence, whether the key word appears in the whole text or just the abstract, and so on. If you widen the search and ask for all entries that have the key word in the whole text, you are likely to be inundated with references. If you are more selective – for example, by requesting keyword entries in the title or abstract – you will limit your search. Also, by adding and combining additional key words, you will further narrow down your search – for example, 'Dementia' and 'Nutrition', or 'Assessment' and 'Mobility'.

How you can plan and search for literature using specific databases

The process of searching for literature is discussed in detail in the partner book in this series, *A Beginner's Guide to Evidence Based Practice in Health and Social Care* by Aveyard, Greenway and Parsons (2023). In this book, we discuss using the acronym **PICOT** to help you identify what you are trying to find out. Each letter prompts you to consider a different aspect of the situation you are seeking information about (Stillwell et al. 2010):

Population
Intervention or issue
Comparison or context
Outcome
Time

* **Population:** who are the people you are interested in investigating with similar characteristics, such as gender, age, condition, problem, location or role? For example, older people in residential care, homeless people, mothers under 45, patients/clients who have had knee replacements, patients/clients who have accessed paramedic services for chest pain, staff who work out of hours, students who access study advice?
* **Intervention/issue:** this could be diagnostic, therapeutic, preventative, exposure, managerial, costs, and so on.
* **Comparison/context:** this can be against another intervention or no intervention. Comparisons can be made against national or professional standards or guidelines. The context of the study might be where the study takes place, such as in a community setting or in a particular country.
* **Outcome:** faster, cheaper, reduction or increase in symptoms, events, episodes, prognosis, mortality, accuracy, etc. For more qualitative research, the outcome may be the perceptions or experience of the participants.
* **Time:** this may or may not be relevant, for example, days post-op or post-intervention, or within 24 hours of accessing the service.

Identifying what you need to find out

* Think critically and carefully about what you want to find out (consider the **PICOT** prompt, or maybe make a spider diagram or list all of the issues).
* Identify your **key words** and use a thesaurus to find alternative words (synonyms). Key words should reflect the topic you are searching for, remembering to use all words, not just popular or current terms. Think widely and laterally!

- There is also the **truncation** or * facility (on some databases this is another symbol – do check!). This enables you to identify all possible endings of the key term you write. To use this, you need to identify the 'root' of the word (i.e. the part of the word that doesn't change) and put the * after the last letter of the root. For example, Disab* will find you *disab*ility, *disab*led and *disab*ilities.
- *Set limits* on the search requested – consider whether you want to limit the number of hits you get by specifying language, date, title or abstract.
- Use Boolean operators. These will help you to refine your search:
  - AND ensures that *each term* you have entered is searched for. This will reduce the number of hits you get, as each term must be included in the article for it to be recognized. Be careful about using too many ANDs, as this may narrow your search too much.
  - OR ensures that *either one term or another* is selected. This will increase the number of hits you get, as you only need to identify one of the terms for the article to be selected. All these words should broadly mean the same thing.
  - NOT enables you to restrict your search, for example 'Hand washing' NOT 'COVID-19' would ensure that a search on hand washing did not identify papers specific to the COVID-19 epidemic.
- Find out how each database operates, as they are all slightly different.

Planning your search

The following key word search table illustrates how you could plan your search using truncated words, and the AND/OR facility.

	1		**2**		**3**
a)	disab* or	AND	attitud* or	AND	student* or
b)	handicap* or		belief* or		learner* or
c)	impair*		valu* or		apprentice*

Setting your limits

You can also specify whether you wish to search throughout *the whole article* for the key word, or whether you want to limit your search to the

abstract or title. This will depend on whether you get too many or too few hits.

- If you limit your search to identifying the key word in the title alone, this might exclude a lot of references that are relevant, because the title may not use the key word you have chosen.
- Conversely, if you search through all the articles for your key word, you may be overwhelmed with literature.

You should therefore consider selecting the abstract, as this gives a brief overview of what the article contains and what type of writing it is.

An abstract is a short summary of what an article is about and usually appears before the introduction. It is often available directly through the subject-specific database even when access to the full article is not. You should be able to tell from the abstract whether it is a research article or not.

Documenting your search strategy

It will be beneficial when producing information for practice or an assignment if you can document *how* you searched for the best available evidence rather than just relying on readily available information. This demonstrates that you took a critical approach to finding your evidence and did not use the first pieces of information that came to hand. The following chart has been developed to help you to do this.

Database	Limits set	Key search terms	Number of hits
Example CINAHL	2013–2023, English language only, word appearing in abstract only	Female* OR women OR woman AND catheter*	251

Remember …

- Searching for literature is time-consuming and is a skill that needs to be developed over time – you are advised not to leave it until the last minute.

- If you do not receive any 'hits' from your search, keep searching with different key words, or you may need to broaden your topic until you identify literature that is linked to your subject area.
- If you get too many hits, you will need to re-focus your search, possibly by date or language.
- Keep a record of the search terms you have used and the results of these searches, and include these in your publication or assignment, perhaps in an appendix.
- Even if you do not find any evidence, this is still a useful 'finding' so long as you can demonstrate that your search has been thorough.

How to find additional evidence that may not be found using databases

Electronic searches of subject-specific databases are not 100 per cent comprehensive and are unlikely to identify all the relevant literature on your topic.

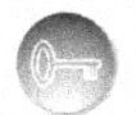

Despite advances in technology, electronic searching is not 100 per cent effective or accurate. This means that you can miss key evidence through electronic searching. The reasons for this are as follows:

- Some relevant literature might have been categorized using different key words and therefore will not be identified by one particular search strategy.
- The topic you are interested in may only be mentioned briefly in papers on broader topics and therefore will not be identified by key words or in the index when these papers are entered onto the database. As a result, they may not be recognized when you search.
- The title of the paper may be misleading, for example, some authors use humorous titles or phrases that you may not be familiar with.

If you want to be really thorough, additional approaches to take when searching for evidence include:

- Looking in the reference lists of the papers you *have* found (this process is called '**snowballing**').
- Looking through the contents pages of back copies of journals that you have previously found useful.

- Asking experts who may have attended conferences or who have access to, as yet, unpublished ideas or contacts.
- Supplementing your search with the more readily available literature, as identified in Chapter 2.
- Searching for papers written by experts in the field.

Do remember, however, that this type of searching should be in addition to your electronic search rather than a substitute for it.

Getting hold of your sources

The references to which you are directed are likely to be found in journals, books and other publications. Books are generally held in a library or bookshop and you will need to access these in person; however, the number of books available electronically in the form of e-books is growing.

Journals can generally be accessed either in person from the library where they are held as hard copies, or online though a library's electronic journals collection. You are strongly advised to become familiar with your electronic library, as most university and workplace libraries provide access to journals in 'full-text' format, meaning you can locate and download many articles without leaving your computer. *You will need a password to access these.* Sometimes there will be a link from the search engine database to the full text article in the electronic library. If you cannot access the journal article you are looking for, you can try Research Gate, where many researchers upload their work, or you can contact the authors directly.

Using abstracts to select the most useful results

Once you have completed a search, you need to consider what type of evidence you have identified on your chosen topic. Depending on the number of hits generated, you probably won't be able to download or access all of the articles and you will need to make sense of what you have found. It is better not to rely on the title alone, as this can be misleading. This is because the focus of the article is often unclear from the title alone. Instead, read the abstract.

Find several different journal papers and look at their abstracts. See if you can tell what type of paper each one is (e.g. a review, a research paper, an opinion piece).

What is the 'best available' evidence?

Once you have found your evidence, you need to consider what type of evidence is most useful to you. In other words, what exactly should you be looking for? You may have heard of the term '**hierarchy of evidence**'. Strong evidence is at the top of the hierarchy and the weakest evidence is at the bottom. Classifications as to what counts as strong evidence vary according to what you are trying to find out, as we will see in the examples later on in this chapter.

In general terms, you will find the **literature review**, in particular the **systematic review**, at the top of the hierarchy of evidence in almost every classification you come across. The systematic review is generally considered to provide the most useful information. A systematic review is a very detailed literature review and seeks to summarize all available evidence on a topic. Less detailed reviews are called literature reviews.

If you come across a systematic review when searching for evidence, you will likely have found the best available evidence for your topic, especially if the review is recent and it is clear that it has been carried out thoroughly. You can probably stop searching and use this review to inform your practice and academic work. Beware of less detailed reviews that have not been undertaken systematically or transparently. These will be less useful to you.

How you can recognize a literature review

Authors of a review will not have conducted their own first-hand study (e.g. experiments or interviews) but instead will have collected together the research of others in order to reach a new conclusion. A good review will tell you how it was undertaken. As discussed in Chapter 2, a good systematic literature review will be written up in the same manner as a research article, with a research or review question, aims and objectives, and a method section outlining how the review was undertaken. The method should tell you how the researchers searched for literature, what literature they included and why, and what they excluded and why. By reading the method, you should have a good idea about how the researchers carried out their literature review. The *conclusion* will be based on weighing up the evidence presented by all the literature reviewed. You may find that a review concludes that the research evidence is strong or that there is insufficient high-quality evidence.

This is just as important for informing our writing and professional practice as a strong positive or negative result from experimental research.

One other point to note is the use of the term 'systematic review'. The term is often used in relation to the Cochrane and Campbell Systematic Reviews as discussed in previous chapters. However, the term is not restricted for use by these review types. You will often find the term used to refer to other types of literature reviews that have been undertaken systematically. This is discussed further in the section below.

Systematic reviews

A **systematic review** is the most detailed type of review. It is undertaken in a rigorous and systematic way and often aims to identify *all* available literature on a topic with clear explanations of the approach taken (methodology).

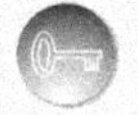

Systematic reviews that have a detailed research methodology should be regarded as a strong form of evidence when they are identified as relevant to a literature review question.

As discussed in Chapter 2, the most common way of conducting a systematic review is through the **Cochrane Collaboration**. The Cochrane Collaboration has a focus on the effectiveness of health care interventions. It's sister organization, the **Campbell Collaboration**, has a focus on social care. On both websites, you can browse by topic for reviews and they have a plain English summary to help you understand complex jargon. Information about the Cochrane Library reviews is available at www.cochrane.org/reviews. Information about the Campbell Library reviews is available at www.campbellcollaboration.org. Some international organizations also present systematic reviews in different languages.

A systematic review undertaken in the detail required by the Cochrane or Campbell Collaboration is usually considered to be the most detailed and robust form of review. For example, in the UK they are used in the formulation of guidelines for the National Institute for Health and Care Excellence (NICE) [http://www.nice.org.uk/]. NICE recommendations for clinical practice are based on the best available evidence. Also, the Centre for Reviews and Dissemination is a useful and reliable source and has a database relating to health policy and practice [http://www.york.ac.uk/inst/crd/]. If you reside in a country other than the UK, you should seek out any national or international guidelines or standards. However, systematic reviews are not only conducted by the Cochrane and Campbell Collaborations. They can be undertaken independently by researchers and can be undertaken to address a range of topics, including qualitative and mixed methods reviews.

Why are systematic reviews so useful?

Systematic literature reviews are important because they seek to:

- Summarize all the literature available on a particular topic.
- Prevent one 'high-profile' piece of information having too much influence.
- Present an analysis of the available literature so that the reader does not have to access each individual research report included in the review.

Limitations of systematic reviews

Systematic reviews are sometimes criticized because they often:

- Include only the highest quality studies, omitting other evidence that might be useful. This does not always relate to qualitative systematic reviews.
- Over-simplify, decontextualize and summarize the evidence to such an extent that the findings are stripped of meaning.

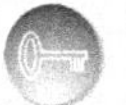

Before you carry out a database search, access one of the websites above that contain systematic reviews and you may save yourself hours of searching other databases.

Descriptive (or narrative) literature reviews

Beware of reviews that have a very brief or no published method informing the reader how the review was carried out. These are sometimes referred to as **narrative** or **descriptive reviews**. Such a review might be no more than a biased or randomly assembled collection of research papers about a given topic. Consequently, the conclusions drawn are likely to be inaccurate.

Although it may refer to a lot of literature or evidence, a narrative literature review does not tell the reader how the authors identified or why they included this literature. You do not know if the writers just 'cherry picked' the literature they wanted to include, ignoring every-thing else. Many papers in health and social care are written in this way. While you might find them useful for information, you should be aware that they will not give you a comprehensive range of information on the topic because they do not state the criteria used to include or exclude information. If you come across an information or discussion article that includes various references and wonder if it is a literature review, look to see if there is a clearly written method section informing you how the information included was identified. If there is no such method section, the article is not strictly a 'literature review' – or at least not a detailed one; instead, it is more likely to be an informative discussion of literature.

What if you cannot find a literature review or systematic review?

If no reviews are available, the next best thing is to access individual pieces of research on a topic. If you have done a thorough and focused search, you will have highlighted the range of research papers that are available on your topic, rather than identifying a single paper simply by flicking through a journal that you have come across. It is important to remember that one individual piece of research – however good it is – is never enough evidence on its own to recommend a change in practice. Thus if you cannot find a review, look at as many research articles as you can on the topic you are interested in. In the absence of a review, these will be your best available evidence.

Research evidence

Recognizing individual research papers and systematic reviews

You can distinguish a research paper from a 'non-research' paper by the way that it is structured. As with a systematic literature review, a research paper will have a research question, stated aims and a method section that tells you how the research was undertaken. This is followed by a results or findings section, a discussion with conclusions and recommendations.

What type of individual research papers should you look for?

In very general terms, research is divided into three types: **qualitative**, **quantitative** and **mixed methods**.

'Mixed methods' approaches use more than one type of research. It is important to consider what type of research will address what you are hoping to find out (this does not matter as much in a literature review, as reviews can contain both qualitative and quantitative papers). The type of research you find is often determined by the type of question you are asking. So you need to *think critically* about this before you start your search. To do this, it is useful to consider the main differences between qualitative and quantitative research.

The main differences between qualitative and quantitative research

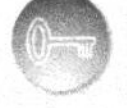

Qualitative research *generally uses interviews to explore the* ***experience*** *or meaning of an issue in depth. The results are presented using* ***words***.

Quantitative research *generally explores if something is* ***effective*** *or not, or measures the* ***amount*** *of something. The results are generally presented using* ***numbers*** *or statistics.*

What is the best type of research?

There is no 'best type' of research. Some topics are best explored using qualitative research and others using quantitative research. To gain a better insight into an issue, mixed methods can be used, thus it is not possible to say which type of research is better in any general sense. There is broad agreement that literature reviews are at the top of the hierarchy of evidence for all situations you can think of, but only if they have been conducted thoroughly. After that, it depends on what you are looking for. You may come across the so-called traditional 'hierarchy of evidence'. This hierarchy applies only when you need to measure the effectiveness of something, for example, does something work or not. If you want to know if something works or is effective, the best way to find out is to test it against something else. This may be a new treatment against the standard treatment. Therefore, if we accept that a systematic review is the strongest evidence to help us answer this question, the next strongest evidence will be the randomized control trial (RCT) – or experiment – because it directly tests one treatment or intervention against another. We discuss RCTs in the section below.

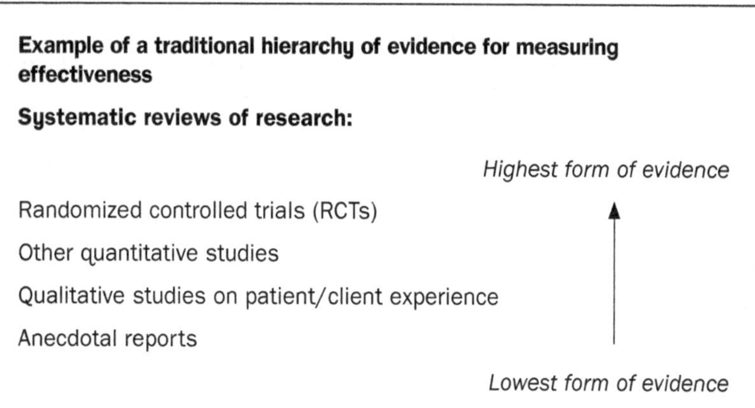

However, do not be misled into thinking that this hierarchy works in all cases. If only things were so simple! It is not the case that the randomized controlled trial is always the next best research design after the systematic literature review. Unfortunately, there is no one hierarchy that works in all cases. While it is probably true that a systematic review will be most useful to you, after that what is most useful depends on what you are hoping to find out. Different situations require different types of evidence. You can see from the discussion of qualitative and quantitative research above that the two approaches are different and give different types of evidence. The hierarchy also suggests that quantitative studies, and in particular RCTs, provide stronger evidence than qualitative studies. However, this is not always the case; it depends what you are trying to find out – you cannot find everything out using an RCT or even quantitative research. For example, if you want to know whether a particular intervention is successful – such as providing day care for children at risk, or using a new type of leg ulcer dressing – you need a study that directly compares one intervention with another: in other words, comparing two types of day care, *or* comparing day care with staying at home, *or* comparing different types of leg ulcer dressings. This would probably be an RCT.

The most common type of study for determining whether an intervention is successful or not is an RCT or a similar quantitative study; so the hierarchy does 'work' on this occasion. However, RCTs would not be useful if you wished to find out about clients' experience of day care or patients' views about a new leg ulcer dressing. A direct comparison of the effectiveness of either day care or dressings will not tell you about what the care or treatment was like for the patient/client. In order to find out about this, you would usually need qualitative research. Therefore, the 'traditional' hierarchy of evidence is only helpful for assessing strength of evidence in certain cases

A rough hierarchy of evidence when looking at patient/client experiences is as follows. In this case, after the systematic literature review, qualitative studies are often most useful in helping us understand the experiences of patients/clients because these studies are designed to obtain in-depth information from participants. We discuss qualitative research in more detail below.

Thus there is no one hierarchy of evidence that works in all situations. Beware of any literature that describes a hierarchy of evidence as if there is *only* one. You should think critically and ask, 'What type of evidence do I need for my question?' It is far better to work out what type of evidence you need for your particular topic and then make up your own 'hierarchy of evidence' for what you are looking for (Aveyard et al. 2023).

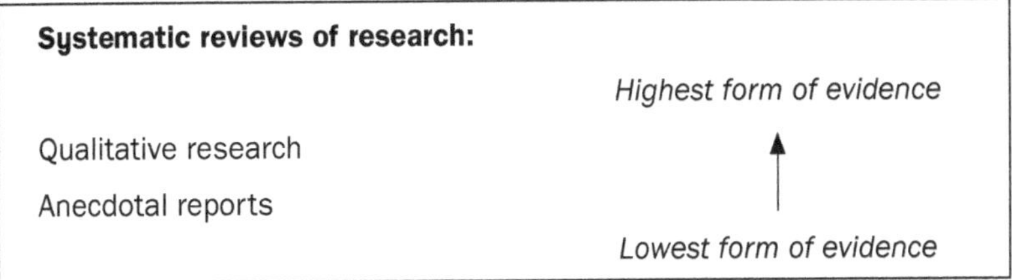

We now provide a brief overview of the characteristics of the main types of research (qualitative and quantitative) followed by some examples.

You are advised to consult additional texts (e.g. Aveyard et al. 2023) to provide you with a more detailed overview of different research methodologies.

Qualitative research

If you are trying to find out about patients' or clients' experiences, such as how they feel about their care, or what it is like to live with a particular condition, then you need to search for qualitative research. This is because qualitative research explores topics through discussion with the people involved, often using interviews or group interviews. Qualitative research is used to explore topics that cannot be measured numerically. For example, the question 'What is it like to move to Italy (or any other country) as a political refugee?' is one that would be answered best by conducting in-depth interviews with the refugees themselves. Qualitative research studies tend to include fewer participants than quantitative studies. Participants in qualitative research are selected because they know about the issue and not at random, as in quantitative studies.

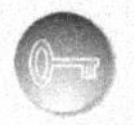

*The aim of all qualitative approaches is to **explore the meaning** of and develop **in-depth understanding** of the research topic as experienced by the participants included in the research.*

There are a wide variety of approaches to qualitative research. You are likely to encounter many different approaches to this type of research when you read the literature. It is useful to be able to recognize these different approaches and to understand why one approach may have been selected for a specific research question. Some are simply described in the literature as 'qualitative studies', while others are named according to the particular qualitative approach that is followed. For example, here are three popular approaches:

- **Grounded theory** is a way of finding out about what happens in a social setting and then making wider generalizations about the way things happen. It is a 'bottom-up' approach in which data are collected, analysed and used to describe the way things happen in social life.
- **Phenomenology** is the study of the 'lived experience' – what it is actually like to live with a particular condition or experience. Phenomenological studies often use in-depth interviews as their means of

data collection, as this allows participants the opportunity to explore and describe their experiences within an interview setting.
- **Ethnography** is the study of human culture. An ethnographic study focuses on a community (i.e. a specific group of people) to gain insight into how its members behave. Observation or participant observation and/or in-depth interviews may be undertaken to achieve this.

Characteristics of qualitative research

- *Depth* rather than breadth is the focus of qualitative research.
- Researchers seek to understand the *whole* of an experience and gain insight into the participants' circumstances.
- The data collected are not numerical but are collected, often through interview, using the *words and descriptions* given by participants.
- Researchers do not set out to look for specific ideas, hoping to confirm pre-existing beliefs. Instead, they code the data according to ideas arising from those data. This process is often referred to as *inductive*.
- There is no use of statistics in qualitative research; the results are *descriptive and interpretative.*
- **Sample** sizes tend to be small. A small sample is required because in-depth understanding (rather than statistical analysis) is sought from the information-rich participants in the study.
- Qualitative studies are not directly generalizable in a statistical sense (see the section on statistics later in this chapter) but their results can be used and interpreted by others. This is sometimes called **transferability**.

Data collection and analysis in qualitative research

In-depth interviews are generally used to collect data. These can be conducted with individuals or 'focus groups'. Qualitative research is useful when you are looking for in-depth answers to questions that cannot be answered in numerical form. The aim of most qualitative data analysis is to study the interview scripts obtained and develop an understanding of the data. The data are organized through coding and themes are then generated from the data set. For this reason, large numbers of participants are rarely used (and are not necessarily appropriate) in qualitative research. Qualitative data can also be collected by questionnaires/surveys when there is space for free text (so people can express their thoughts and feelings).

The data are generally analysed using the words of the original interview transcripts. The findings or results are then coded and written up as themes, which describe the main findings. Researchers usually provide examples of quotes from their participants in the write-up of their findings. The results of such research are not usually presented numerically or statistically, and the findings are not generalizable to other situations, individuals or groups – that is, predictions about the wider population cannot be made from the results of a small study. However, the results of qualitative studies are 'stand-alone' in the sense that the reader can transfer the findings of a study to help make sense of other comparable situations. What is important in a qualitative study is that the process used to undertake it is transparent. The relationship between the participants and researchers should be described together with other factors that influenced the findings, such as the skill of the interviewer and location of the interviews.

How can you identify a good qualitative study?

In addition to the '**Six questions for critical thinking**', you might also find it useful to use a critical appraisal tool that is specifically intended for use with qualitative studies, such as the Critical Appraisal Skills Programme (CASP). This is a qualitative research appraisal tool, one of many such tools available at http://www.caspinternational. org/?o=1012.

Remember that well-designed qualitative studies produce better data than poorly designed studies. Do not be put off by a small sample size – qualitative studies tend to be small. You would expect to read details of how the study was carried out and, if interviews were conducted, how these were transcribed and analysed.

Quantitative research

If you are researching aspects of health or social care that you can measure directly, such as comparing the healing rate of a wound or recovery after an injury, then you will need quantitative research. This is because quantitative research (sometimes called positivist research) uses numerical measurement to explore research questions. For example, the question 'Does nicotine replacement therapy help people stop smoking?'

can be answered numerically by counting the number of people who stop smoking when using nicotine replacement therapy versus those who do not. Quantitative research studies tend to involve larger numbers of participants who are often selected at random.

If you wish to find out about the effectiveness of – or comparison between – treatments or interventions that can be directly measured or counted, then you need to look for quantitative research. 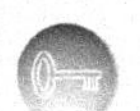

Approaches used in quantitative research

- **Randomized controlled trials.** Quantitative **experimental** methods can be used to measure the *effectiveness of an intervention* (in other words, studies that find out whether a specific intervention really works). The most rigorous form of study is the randomized control trial (RCT). Such a trial can be used to test the effectiveness of many care or treatment options where it is permissible and ethical to randomly divide the sample group and monitor the outcome. In an RCT, participants are allocated at random into two or more groups – this is called **randomization**. An intervention is then given to only one of the groups and the outcomes in the different groups are compared. One can then look at the differences between the groups at the end of the study and see whether those who received an intervention fared better than those who did not. This is really the only way to tell whether an intervention is effective.
- **Other experimental methods.** It is not always possible to undertake an RCT because care or treatment cannot be withheld from individuals in one group. Other quantitative research methods can be used for experimental research designs that are not RCTs. These are often called 'quasi experiments' because they are not carried out in the form of a true experiment (or RCT). Other types of studies are **cohort studies** and **case control studies**. These are studies that try to link the causes of diseases and/or interventions and/or social situations. Cohort studies and case control studies were first used to observe the effects of an exposure (e.g. smoking) on the health of those observed.
- **Questionnaires and surveys**. These are studies in which a sample is taken at *any one point in time* from *a defined group of people* and observed/assessed. These studies tend to be quantitative, as it can be difficult to get good descriptive data from a questionnaire.

Questionnaires and surveys are useful when looking for evidence about the prevalence of a particular event or when requiring information about a large group of people. Remember that studies based on questionnaires and surveys have many limitations, as outlined below, and their results should be viewed with caution. Electronic sources such as email are increasingly being used as a cheaper and more accessible format for questionnaires/surveys.

Characteristics of quantitative research

- Quantitative studies use methods of data collection that involve *measuring*: size, amount, scales, frequency (e.g. how many?, how much?, how often?).
- They try to be *objective*.
- Data are analysed using *statistical tests* and results are presented using *numbers*.
- The studies tend to be *large* and involve many participants so that the findings can be applied in other contexts. This is called **generalizability**.

Data collection and analysis in quantitative research

Data are generally collected in numerical form, such as how many people responded to a particular drug or type of exercise. The results of quantitative research are usually presented using numbers or statistics. Sometimes it is really hard to understand the statistics and tables in quantitative research but there are a few key things you should be able to understand. Researchers themselves sometimes employ statisticians to help them analyse and interpret results.

When you next look at a quantitative research study, read the discussion where the results are explained and then go back to the actual numbers to see if you can understand them better.

Quantitative data are often presented as statistics. There are two types of statistics: descriptive and inferential.

Descriptive statistics describe the data or results in a paper. These statistics should describe clearly the main results, for example, how many people answered 'yes' to a particular question, or the most common response to a question. Let's take the example of the efforts that are being made to reduce neonatal mortality in Sub-Saharan Africa. Zegeye et al. (2022) explored whether the widespread use of skilled birth attendants in Guinea had any effect on neonatal mortality and child and maternal health. This was clearly a quantitative study, as mortality rates and other health outcomes can be counted. The researchers undertook a look-back exercise in Guinea in which the use of skilled birth attendants (SBA) was analysed and correlated to neonatal mortality (NMR) and other outcomes for the mother and baby. Data from 14,402 births that had been attended by a skilled birthing attendant were analysed according to income and education of the mother and also against births where an attendant had not been present. Amongst other findings they reported the demographic information about the women attended by the skilled birth attendants:

A total of 14,402 participants for SBA and 39,348 for NMR were involved in this study. Out of the SBA sample, 10,514 women (73.0%) were rural residents. Regarding maternal educational level, 11,554 (80.2%) had no formal education, only 1565 (10.9%) had primary school and 1282 (8.9%) had secondary or higher education.

(Zegeye et al. 2022: 5)

You can see that these results present a **description** of the results *in that particular study* only. They do not tell us about the demographic information of the women attended to by skilled birth attendants across Guinea as a whole. However, these descriptive results are important as they tell us exactly what the study found. The research should be clearly presented and you should be able to ascertain easily what the results of the study were.

Inferential statistics are used to make predictions. Once we have a detailed description of an event (the more or the bigger the better; we would not be very confident in the results of a comparison of one trained birth attendant and one untrained attendant), we can use the results of statistical tests to make predictions about the outcome of other similar events. We do this all the time in sport. If you follow a particular sport, you will have noted that commentators make predictions about who is going to win. These predictions are based on many observations of who won on previous occasions. Although we cannot tell if an individual or team will win again, if we have enough prior evidence to go on, we can make a reasonable prediction. This is what statisticians do. They look at what has happened in a particular event (such as in a study situation) and they then make a prediction as to whether we are likely to see this result outside the research setting. The better the data they have to work from, the better the predictions they can make.

In other words, statistics can tell us how likely it would be for the findings from Zegeye and colleagues' study to be found in a larger population. From these statistics we can then make generalizations about whether the results of the study are applicable more widely. You can see why this is important.

When predictions are made about what is likely to happen in a larger population (not the sample used) on the basis of the findings of a study, we call this making inference or using inferential statistics. In other words, statisticians try to determine the extent to which the data obtained from a sample is reflective of the wider population as a whole. They tell us what might be expected to happen in the wider population. In simple terms, the bigger the sample, the more certain you can be that the sample prevalence is close to the population prevalence. In other words, if the sample size in the research is large, it is more likely it can be applied to the whole population. For example, if you have a questionnaire survey of 1000 people from around the country, of which 500 stated a preference for holidaying abroad, inferential statistics can be used to determine whether this result would be likely to be accurate for the whole population. But if the sample size was 50, it would be less likely that the results would represent national views.

When you read a quantitative research paper, these ideas can be expressed in a range of statistical terms, including (but not limited to) **confidence intervals** and/or as **p values**. Confidence intervals reflect the confidence we can have that the sample is an accurate indication of the true population prevalence. In addition to confidence intervals, you might find probability expressed as a **p value** (or probability). The p value expresses the probability of the results shown in the paper being due to chance. It is important to determine the likelihood that the findings are down to chance or whether they reflect what happened in the research.

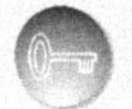

The lower the p value, the less likely it is that the occurrence is due to chance. If a p value is less than 0.05 (1:20), we say the occurrence is unlikely to be due to chance. If the p value is say, 0.5, we would say that 50% of the time the occurrence would be due to chance and therefore not likely to be due to the intervention in question.

Zegeye et al. do not report p values and confidence intervals but use other statistics to demonstrate how generalizable their findings are:

We found significant absolute and relative wealth-driven inequality in SBA in Guinea from 1999 to 2016 using simple (D, R) and complex (PAR, PAF) measures.

(2022: 5)

It is not necessary that you understand all the statistics used within a research paper but it is important that you understand that these statistics are used to make generalizations beyond the sample in the study. This is indicated by use of the term 'significant'. This is the main purpose of quantitative research.

In their study of birth attendants, Zegeye et al. (2022) did not calculate p values. If they had, however, the values would tell us how likely it was that the difference between the outcomes in the two groups (those who had trained birth attendants and those who did not) was due to chance or was really due to the training of the birth attendants. Even if both groups had trained birth attendants, you would likely see a variety of outcomes in the two groups due to natural differences between them. This could possibly be a chance variation, as no two groups are ever exactly the same, or it could be due to the intervention. What we want to determine is whether the difference between those cared for by the trained birth attendants and those cared for in the traditional manner can be attributed to the training of the birth attendant or whether it is just a chance finding. The p value can then be calculated to determine whether the differences in outcomes observed is due to chance or not.

To calculate the p value we use the **null hypothesis**. This is a phrase that is used when you state (in order to test it) that there is no relationship between the different elements (or variables) under study. This can be calculated using a statistical test, such as the chi-squared test. A p value of 0.05, for example, means that there is a 1:20 chance of seeing these results if the null hypothesis were true, and is not generally low enough to rule out chance.

Let's imagine that Zegeye et al. (2022) found a p value of 0.002. This would mean that there is a 2:1000 chance that the differences were due to chance alone. A p value expressed as $p = 0.002$ indicates that it is unlikely that the improvement in risk reduction in the women attended to by the trained birth attendant was due to chance.

Here we have provided a brief overview of the commonly held beliefs about and ways of presenting inferential statistics. Some people find these concepts easy to comprehend; others find it more difficult and need to read and re-read the points made several times before they begin to make sense. If this applies to you, then do re-read the section above. You might also find it useful to consult other texts that describe the use of statistics. For those who find the concepts easy to follow, consider developing your understanding through further reading of books on statistics that are specifically designed for health and social care professionals.

How can you identify a good quantitative study?

In addition to the '**Six questions for critical thinking**', you might also find it useful to use a critical appraisal tool that is specifically intended for use with quantitative studies, such as the Critical Appraisal Skills Programme (CASP). This is a qualitative research appraisal tool, one of many such tools available at http://www.caspinternational. org/?o=1012.

Remember that poorly designed quantitative studies produce weak data. To know if a study has been carried out well, you need to know the method used. In general, the study will be more reliable if the sample size is large, the results are statistically significant and the method of study is appropriate to its aims and well described.

Some examples of qualitative and quantitative research

It is important to be clear in your mind about the differences between qualitative and quantitative research. To get you used to thinking about the differences, we provide some examples of topics you might want to find out about. Read each example carefully and decide whether you would be looking for qualitative or quantitative research to address the topic. The answers are given below.

*Looking at the **example questions** below, decide which approach is best – qualitative or quantitative? Or maybe a mixture of the two (mixed methods)?*

- What are the experiences of single parenthood in an inner city?
- What types of illegal drugs are used by people aged between 18 and 21?
- Do antibiotics shorten the length of an episode of tonsillitis?
- Which factors lead to a student's decision to leave university in their first year?
- Which universities have the highest attrition rates?
- Why do patients/clients prefer 'single-sex' wards?

The example questions and some possible research approaches

What are the experiences of single parents in an inner city?
You would be looking for qualitative research because this information is likely to be obtained through in-depth interviews exploring the experiences of single parents in detail.

What types of illegal drugs are used by people aged between 18 and 21?
You would be looking for quantitative research because this information can be measured numerically – that is, the types of drugs and who takes them can be measured. Whether it is possible to get an accurate answer to these questions is another matter!

Do antibiotics shorten the length of an episode of tonsillitis?
Again, this would be explored using quantitative research because this information can be measured numerically. In this case, you can measure the length of an illness and then find out whether the person had taken antibiotics or not.

Which factors lead to a student's decision to leave university in their first year?
This is not a question that can be easily considered using exact numerical measurement. This is because the information is not easily quantifiable. The information is likely to be collected using in-depth interviews and therefore using a qualitative approach. However, you may also find that a mixed methods approach is useful here as students might be able to rank their reasons for leaving university on a questionnaire.

Which universities have the highest attrition rates?
This question can be easily answered using quantitative methods – attrition rates are straightforward to measure and can be counted.

> This contrasts with the question above, which necessitates a mixed methods or qualitative approach.
>
> *Why do patients/clients prefer 'single-sex' wards?*
> This question requires a qualitative approach to research because the focus is on the reasons for patients'/clients' preferences (this question assumes that we already know about patients'/clients' preferences). Note, however, that if the question were simply 'Do patients/clients prefer "single-sex" wards?', then a quantitative approach could be used.

 *Next time you come across some research, try and read around the type of research it is, so you can more easily understand the approach. You can use research textbooks and glossaries such as* http://www.cochrane.org/glossary *to help you.*

Many broad topic areas can be explored using both qualitative and quantitative approaches; it depends which aspect of the topic you are focusing on or want to explore. Take the following three topics and consider how each *could* be explored using either a qualitative or quantitative approach (we offer some suggestions below):

1. Diabetes
2. Young carers
3. Binge drinking in teenagers

Qualitative research questions:

1. What is an adult pregnant woman's experience of living with diabetes?
2. What is it like to be a young carer?
3. Why has the incidence of binge drinking escalated in recent years?

Quantitative research questions:

1. Which drug is most effective in managing diabetes?
2. How many young carers are there in Western Australia?
3. At what age do people who binge drink start drinking?

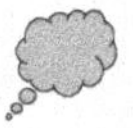

Think critically about how, depending on the question being asked, some aspects of a topic are best explored using a quantitative approach and some a qualitative approach.

Once you have grasped these main types of research, begin thinking more deeply about the specific type of information/evidence you would be looking for if you were conducting a search on one of the above topics. This will help you to be more selective about what will be useful for your academic writing or your professional practice. These concepts can be difficult to understand, especially if you are new to thinking and reading about research, and refining these concepts further can be confusing. If this is the case, then you may want to re-focus on more simple considerations such as whether the research you require is qualitative or quantitative.

Will you always find up-to-date research and information for your practice?

While there has been a marked increase in the amount of available information, it is still the case that some areas of health and social care are under-researched or the research is not of high quality. Research is still developing in some fields, and not all areas of health and social care are underpinned by a sound body of knowledge. So you might find yourself in one of two situations – either:

- you are bombarded by a wealth of information that you need to make sense of, or
- you do not find any information, or only poor quality information that relates to your selected topic.

If you can find a systematic review on your topic, then you have probably identified the best available evidence. Failing that, the next best thing is to collate the available research evidence on your topic. If no research can be identified, then guidelines or policy may help and if these are not available, then professional and expert opinion should be drawn on. Although finding evidence is very important, sometimes there is no specific evidence for what we need and we have to rely on experience and common sense.

The following abstract from Smith and Pell (2003), taken from a Christmas edition of the *British Medical Journal*, and written somewhat in jest (we think!), illustrates this point perfectly (and also demonstrates the process of undertaking a systematic review).

Abstract

Objectives: To determine whether parachutes are effective in preventing major trauma related to gravitational challenge.

Design: Systematic review of randomised controlled trials.

Data sources: Medline, Web of Science, Embase, and the Cochrane Library databases; appropriate internet sites and citation lists.

Study selection: Studies showing the effects of using a parachute during free fall. Main outcome measure death or major trauma, defined as an injury severity score > 15.

Results: We were unable to identify any randomised controlled trials of parachute intervention.

Conclusions: As with many interventions intended to prevent ill health, the effectiveness of parachutes has not been subjected to rigorous evaluation by using randomised controlled trials. Advocates of evidence-based medicine have criticised the adoption of interventions evaluated by using only observational data. We think that everyone might benefit if the most radical protagonists of evidence-based medicine organised and participated in a double blind, randomised, placebo controlled, crossover trial of the parachute.

(Smith and Pell 2003)

We acknowledge that this research paper, in addition to being rather dated, is presented in jest. However it makes a very valid point. This is that good quality evidence will not always be available: you will not always find evidence that is relevant to the care you need to give and this should not stop you carrying out care that is based on common sense or observations that if you jump from an aeroplane without a parachute, you are likely to suffer serious injury!

In summary

To adopt a critical approach to accessing the best available evidence, you need to think about how you can find high-quality, relevant evidence rather than relying solely on readily available evidence. To do this you need to search effectively and this is a skill that takes time to develop. You need to be clear about what you need to find out. You also need to develop skill in understanding the different types of research. We suggest you look for literature reviews and systematic reviews in the first instance, as these will summarize the available evidence. If there are no reviews, then look for available research that has been done on your topic and collate all that is available. You need to think carefully about the type of research that is most useful to you and consider whether you are looking for qualitative, quantitative or mixed methods approaches. We suggest that you get used to thinking critically about the type of research that is most useful to you. Try to follow what is going on in the research, rather than just relying on a summary or abstract. If you cannot identify any research, then draw on professional and expert opinion and other sources.

Key points

1   You need to understand when you need to dig deeper for more or better quality evidence.
2   You will find the best available evidence by conducting a thorough and systematic search.
3   Look for literature reviews or systematic reviews in the first instance.
4   If you do not find a review paper, look for research papers.
5   Identify the type of research that will best address your question.
6   Consider what information will be most useful to you if there is no research evidence.
7   Finally, look for professional or expert opinion if there is no current research.

4 Demonstrating your critical thinking skills in your written work and presentations

- *Why it is important to incorporate critical thinking into your writing and presentations*
- *When you need to incorporate critical thinking into your writing and presentations*
- *How you can develop good critical writing and presentations*
- *The importance of planning your work*
- *The importance of developing a clear, logical and thorough approach to your work*
- *Using different styles of writing and presenting*
- *An example of applying critical thinking skills to written academic work*

> - *Demonstrating critical thinking in verbal presentations*
> - *A checklist for assessing your critical thinking in written work and presentations*
> - *In summary*
> - *Key points*

In this chapter, we will:

- Discuss why it is important to incorporate critical thinking into your writing and presentations (including examined oral presentations and vivas).
- Discuss how you can recognize good critical writing and presentations.
- Identify when you need to incorporate critical thinking into your writing and presentations.
- Explain how you can plan your written work and presentations effectively.
- Discuss how you can present your critical thinking skills effectively in your writing and presentations.

In Chapter 1, we discussed why critical thinking is important for academic work and ultimately for your professional practice. In Chapters 2 and 3, we discussed why it is important to find the best available evidence on a topic, and to think critically about what we read, see and hear. In this chapter, we explore how to demonstrate these skills in your writing and presentations.

Why it is important to incorporate critical thinking into your writing and presentations

You need to be able to communicate your ideas effectively both in writing and verbally. Showing that you have a critical approach to what you read, see and hear will greatly enhance the quality of your work, and will improve your grades. It will also help you to demonstrate that you are a credible practitioner. Using a critical approach will also lead you to develop your ideas and practice, ultimately leading to significant, positive changes in client care. In your professional life, critical thinking is also essential for influencing changes in practice, policies and guidelines.

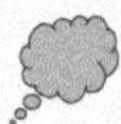

Reflect on why it is important for you to be able to demonstrate your critical thinking and appraisal skills in your writing and verbal presentations.

In both your writing and verbal presentations, you need to show that you have accessed the best available evidence and questioned and analysed what you have read, seen or heard, rather than accepted it at face value. You can achieve this by demonstrating that you understand the information or evidence you use, rather than just reporting it and saying no more about it. This will give your work greater authority.

In your academic work and your professional role, you will need to express your ideas and arguments both in writing and verbally, demonstrating that you are well informed, able to identify relevant information/evidence and appraise the sources of information/evidence that you come across.

A much higher level of skill is therefore needed for critical writing and presenting than that needed for purely descriptive writing and presenting. This is often reflected in grading criteria, particularly once you move into higher levels of study. You are likely to be awarded higher grades if you clearly demonstrate your skills of critical thinking within your work. In this chapter, we explain how you can do that most effectively.

When you need to incorporate critical thinking into your writing and presentations

There are various reasons why you may need to write information or present it verbally, whether as a student or in your professional life within health and social care.

Written information

There are a variety of reasons why you might need to prepare written information, including:

- Academic essays or assignments.
- **Dissertations**, theses or research projects.
- Case studies.
- Reflective diaries or journals.
- Reports for a variety of purposes, including:
  - Research reports, such as those relating to a particular event, issue, aspect of care, intervention or treatment.
  - Incident reports and statements.
- Presenting and justifying recommendations regarding appropriate interventions for the care of a client.
- Policies or guidelines.
- Care plans or care pathways.
- Quality documentation and audits.

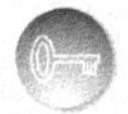

The importance of skilfully crafted, knowledgeable critical writing should not be underestimated – the ability to argue a case in writing can be the key to high-quality, professionally accountable practice and can lead to positive, creative developments in health and social care.

Verbal presentations

There are also a variety of reasons why you might need to prepare and deliver a verbal presentation, including:

- Presenting a case study of a patient/client/family/incident to your colleagues.
- Giving a presentation for an academic assignment.
- Presenting a viva for a dissertation or thesis.
- Giving a teaching session or sharing new information/evidence with colleagues in practice.
- You may also need to present your skills of critical thinking in less formal situations, such as when debating an issue with colleagues, or reflecting on an incident with others – this will be discussed in Chapter 5.

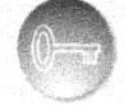

Getting your ideas across in a presentation is just as important as when you write them down. Don't miss the opportunity to demonstrate your skills of critical thinking in your presentations.

How you can develop good critical writing and presentations

Demonstrating skills of critical thinking through your writing or your presentations is something that can be learned and developed. You need to show that you can:

- Select the best available information/evidence.
- Critically appraise these sources.
- Make critical notes based on your reading and critical appraisal.
- Form a clear and logical argument.
- Challenge your own assumptions and broaden your perspectives.

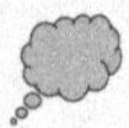

Have you ever come across a speaker or writer who was able to demonstrate their skills of critical thinking clearly? Jot down what you noticed about the way they presented their ideas.

To demonstrate your critical thinking skills in your writing and presentations:

- Your writing should be clearly expressed and logically ordered.
- You should present the best available evidence on a topic, issue or question in a balanced way.
- You need to show that you have assessed and evaluated information, evidence, viewpoints and/or arguments carefully, with a cautious and sceptical approach. Don't assume that all of the ideas or views that you have read or heard are necessarily correct or well founded.
- You should give a well-balanced presentation of what you think of different ideas/viewpoints/arguments/conclusions.
- As well as the above, it is important to acknowledge the limitations of your own ideas and conclusions.

Wellington et al. (2005: 84) suggested that good critical writing (and we think this also applies to presentations) should include the following features:

- *Healthy scepticism ... but not cynicism;*
- *Confidence ... but not 'cockiness' or arrogance;*
- *Judgement which is critical ... but not dismissive;*
- *Opinions ... without being opinionated;*

> - *Having a voice … without 'sounding off';*
> - *Careful evaluation of published work;*
> - *Being 'fair': assessing fairly the strengths and weaknesses of other people's ideas and writing … without prejudice;*
> - *Having your own standpoint and values with respect to an argument, research project or publication … without getting on a soap box;*
> - *Making judgements on the basis of considerable thought and all the available evidence … as opposed to assertions without reason;*
> - *Putting forward recommendations and conclusions, whilst recognising their limitations.*

Later in this chapter, we will provide some tips and strategies for how you can demonstrate these features in your own work.

The importance of planning your work

In order to demonstrate your skills of critical thinking, planning is essential.

Think about the last time you had to write a professional or academic document or an assignment, whether a written piece of work or a verbal presentation. Use the questions below to help you reflect on how you planned for your work. 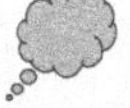

- Were you clear in your aims and focus for your work?
- How did you carry out research into your topic?
- Did you consult anybody for advice or ideas? If so, who?
- Did you access any new information/evidence?
- How confident were you in putting together your work?
- Were you able to express your ideas clearly and logically?
- Did you come across any new ideas or perspectives while preparing your work? If so, did you incorporate these into your work in any way?

The strategies in **bold italics** in the think bubbles in Figure 4.1 reflect a planned and strategic approach. Adopting an unplanned and haphazard approach to preparing your writing or presentations makes you

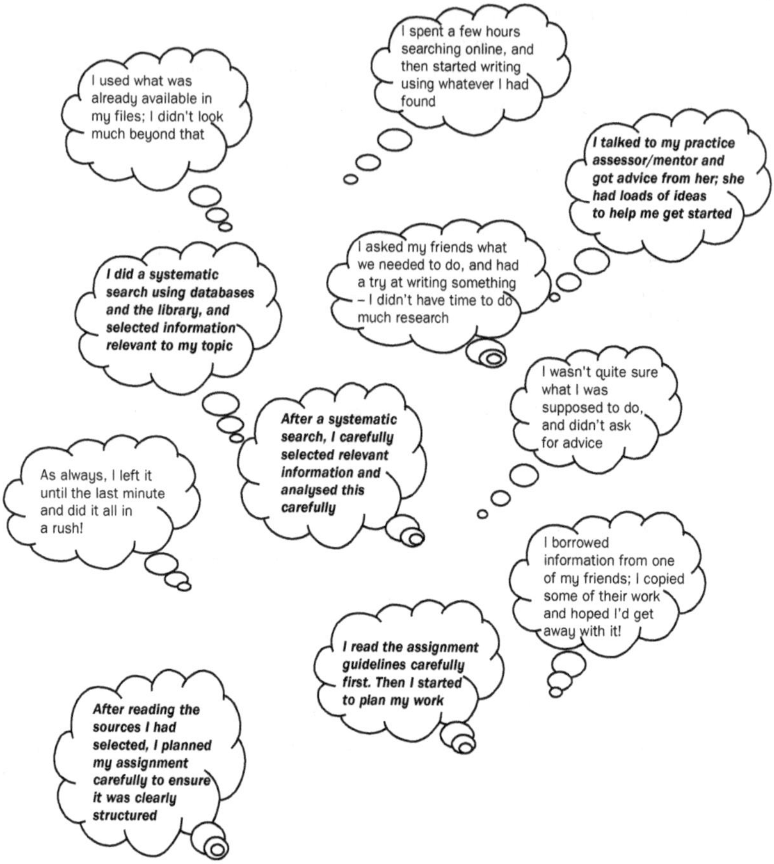

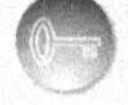

Figure 4.1 Strategies for preparing for an assignment or project

less likely to think critically about what you write. As a result, you are less likely to demonstrate your critical thinking skills clearly and effectively within your work.

You will be more able to adopt a critical approach if you plan your work effectively before you start to work on your assignment, presentation or project. Investing some time in researching and in thinking carefully before you write or present your ideas will pay dividends.

Some 'top tips' to help you prepare your work

Make sure you know exactly what it is that you need to do. Look at the question and/or guidance you have been given, and read it thoroughly. Underline any key words that help you identify your approach (e.g. *Discuss*, *Critically analyse*, *Reflect*, *Report*, *Identify*, *Explore*, etc. We will give examples of these later in the chapter).

Reflect on what you already know, have experienced or think about the topic. Do you have any preconceived views or assumptions that could either inform or influence your approach?

Look at the marking criteria if your work is to be formally assessed. This will help you find out what the markers are looking for when they assess your work, including the skills of critical thinking they hope they will find in your writing or your presentation. You could even add these to a cue column if you are using the Cornell method of note-taking (discussed later in this chapter). If you have been asked to do something on a more informal basis (e.g. writing a report or a set of guidelines, or presenting a brief report), try to **get clear instructions and guidance**, in writing, regarding exactly what is required – this way there is less room for misinterpreting what is expected of you.

Carry out a thorough search for the best available evidence, as discussed in Chapter 3. Select a **range** of **relevant** and **high-quality** information/evidence that will enable you to offer a **balanced, well-informed** argument within your work.

Read the information/evidence carefully. Use the '**Six questions for critical thinking**' (see Chapter 1) to help you think critically about all the sources of information/evidence you have found. Use a framework such as Cornell note-taking (Walter and Owens 2013) to take critical and meaningful notes based on your reading

If you are unsure what to do for any form of assignment or project, seek advice.

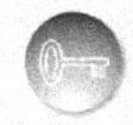

Consider new and alternative perspectives on your topic area – don't dismiss a source if it seems to you to be controversial in its perspectives, or if you disagree with it. Instead, find further evidence to develop your discussion.

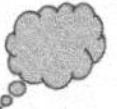

The Cornell note-taking system (Walter and Owens 2013) helps students take notes during their lectures or from their reading in a flexible yet systematic, thoughtful and practical way. The system advises you to take a pre-preparatory approach by dividing a page into three, whether in a handwritten notebook or on an electronic device. The divisions consist of an approximate 6-cm cue column on the left-hand side of the page and a 5-cm horizontal space at the bottom to contain an overall summary (see Figure 4.2 for an example of how to compose a Cornell Note). The main area on the right is where you take notes in your own words, which you can write as bullet points based on your participation in lectures or reading from books or journals. Initially, the cue and summary areas should remain empty. When you reflect on and review your notes, you may return to the cue area to clarify concepts, definitions or reveal relationships

Cues	A national survey of nurse practitioners' patient satisfaction outcomes (Kippenbrock et al. 2019)
What is it?	The paper reports a survey study comparing patient satisfaction with consulting between four professional care providers. The findings suggest that although patients most frequently consult with medical doctors, their satisfaction rates with nurse practitioner consultations are significantly higher compared with medical doctors, physician assistants or osteopaths. The findings are relevant for helping me understand how nurses with advanced practice skills deliver patient-centred care.
Where did you find it?	I undertook a PubMed search through the university library databases.
Who has said this?	The study's six authors were nursing faculty from three US university nursing schools with research interests in nurse practitioner care to underserved patient populations.
When was this written?	The paper was published in 2019, based on retrospective survey data collected in 2018.
Why has this been written?	To provide insight into how patients perceive patient-centred care and consumer choice, to inform health care policymakers about the factors influencing high-quality care.
How do you know if it is of good quality?	The researchers used secondary data, i.e. data collected previously but through a validated tool for measuring consumer satisfaction with health care providers. The sample was predominantly female (61.8%), covering most regions of the USA, and the survey included items on clinician communication, such as listening, information-giving and perceived knowledge of the patient, demonstration of respect and providing opportunities to share decision-making on the benefits of taking or not taking medication. The statistical descriptive analyses showed overall satisfaction with all providers with significantly higher ratings for nurse practitioner consultations. A shortcoming of the study is that medical doctor consultations were disproportionately higher than other providers. Therefore, to convince myself of the significance of research in the field, I will need to look at similar studies with larger sample sizes representing nurse practitioners. US health provision may be context-specific, so looking at similar studies from different international contexts would be helpful.
Summary: *(So what?)* The paper raises the possibility that patients may be more satisfied with nurse practitioner consultations than with other clinicians because nurse practitioners are perceived to be more patient-centred concerning communication, information giving, respect and involving the patient in decision-making; however, more evidence is needed to support these initial claims.	

Figure 4.2 Cornell Note template

between ideas. Alternatively, as suggested in this book, you may draw on some or all of the '**Six questions for critical thinking**' to create cues and enable your note-taking to become a critical tool that you can subsequently draw on for writing your presentations and assignments. The summary area of a Cornell Note is where you write an overall summary of the main point that has impacted your thinking and understanding, such as the '**So what?**' point of the '**Six questions for critical thinking**'.

Drawing a spider diagram (also known as a mind map) is another tool that may help as you prepare and develop your work. For example, look at the simple spider diagram here reproduced in Figure 4.3, put together

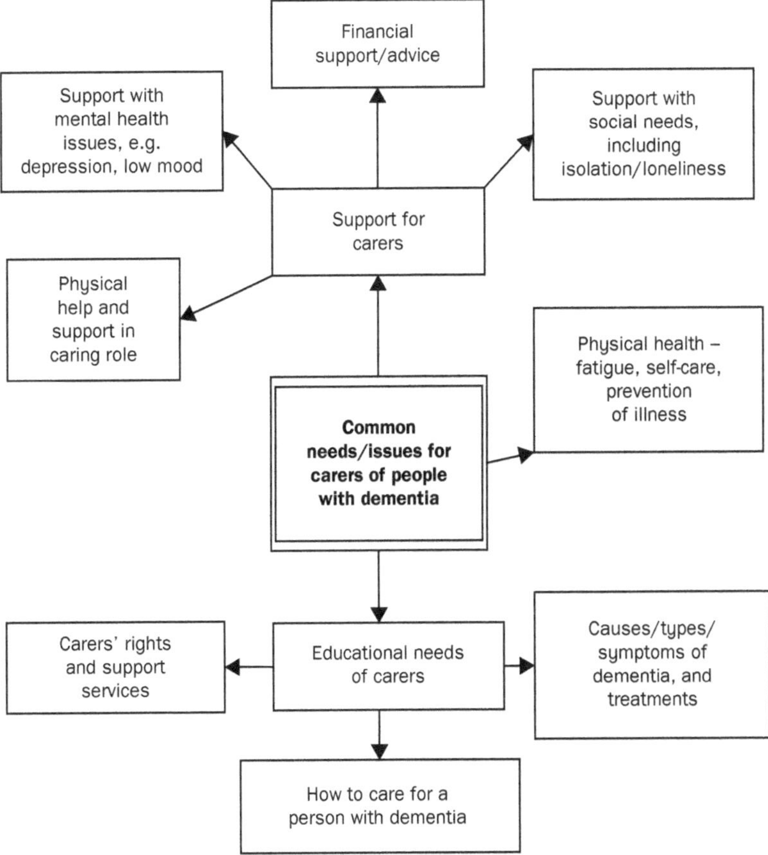

Figure 4.3 A spider diagram

by a student preparing for a presentation about the needs of carers of people with dementia.

Completing a diagram like this could help you identify a clear focus for your work, and different sub-themes that need to be explored. You could extend the diagram further and use this to help you plan your research on the different sub-themes, and how you will focus and structure your writing. A variety of free mind mapping tools are widely available [see, for example, https://www.text2mindmap.com/].

The key point about using tools such as Cornell note-taking, or spider diagrams, is that your note-taking is critical and systematic and can be drawn upon when you come to write your assignments and help you to demonstrate a critical voice within your writing.

The importance of developing a clear, logical and thorough approach to your work

The following nine strategies will help ensure a clear, logical and thorough approach, which will help you demonstrate critical thinking within your written work (more detail is given below):

1. Ensure your focus is clear.
2. Use simple language and clear structure.
3. Use meta-commentary.
4. Demonstrate your use of the best available information/evidence.
5. Use your own words rather than direct quotes from authors (avoiding plagiarism).
6. Demonstrate your skills of critical appraisal and critical analysis.
7. Highlight alternative viewpoints.
8. Bring your points together (synthesize).
9. Summarize and conclude your work effectively.

1. Ensure your focus is clear

You need to ensure that your audience/reader knows what the topic and/ or focus is at the very beginning of your presentation or piece of work. You therefore need to *set out your aims and objectives clearly* – and the words that you use to do this will indicate the level of critical thinking in your presentation. For example:

- *Describe, list* and *identify* – all of these are descriptive and, if not developed further, indicate a low level of critical thinking.
- *Analyse, appraise* and *synthesize* and, where appropriate, *reflect* – all of these demonstrate higher levels of critical thinking.

In the following example, a student clearly outlines the aims and focus of their work.

Example

In this presentation, I will identify the causes of malaria. I will critically analyse the epidemiology of this disease, focusing particularly on those at risk of the disease who live in Latin America. I will then reflect on the implications of my findings for my work in my elective placement next year.

2. Use simple language and clear structure

Sometimes the best writing and presentations are written in plain and simple language. The author or speaker does not try to impress by using complicated words or expressions. It is good to aim to use clear and concise language. You can achieve this by expressing your ideas simply, clearly and logically. You should also explain any complex terms and state what abbreviations mean. Make sure you use profession-specific and up-to-date definitions of key terms. For more complex ideas or concepts, you may need to use several definitions and compare/contrast them.

In your writing, it is essential to understand how to present ideas logically to guide and signpost the reader. Your critical thinking is enhanced with attention to the craft of writing. A helpful way to plan and think about your writing process is by attending to the purposes of sentences, paragraphs, sections, introductions and conclusions.

A sentence represents a single thought and consists of a subject (i.e. 'the nurse'), an object (i.e. the textbook) and a verb or 'doing' word (i.e. to read): *The nurse is reading a textbook.* Sentences can become complex when they deal with two or more ideas. A paragraph is a single set of ideas on one topic. A paragraph starts with a topic sentence introducing the main idea, which may be an introductory paragraph or link to the previous paragraph to develop an idea or a point. The following sentence in the paragraph may provide evidence, an explanation or a definition; this is where you can draw on your critical reading and notes. The following sentence may allow you to offer your evaluation and perspective on the ideas within the paragraph and, once again, could be based on your critical thinking. Finally, it would help if you concluded your paragraph effectively; often, this can be a sentence leading to the next paragraph's topic.

Example

The critical appraisal process revealed two study design approaches. **(Topic)** *Firstly, evaluation studies (n=21) and secondly, qualitative research designs (n= 9)* **(Explanation)** *An evaluation study judges the worth, merit, value, efficacy, impact and effectiveness, whereas research contributes to and extends knowledge (Cohen et al., 2018).* **(Evidence)** *Including evaluation studies in the literature review was vital because it is the most common approach for investigating academic research writing group interventions for nurses.* **(Evaluation)** *In keeping with the rationale for a meta-narrative approach, it conveys how investigations into writing group interventions have unfolded in the discipline.* **(Conclusion)**

Sections of a written paper or assignment are sets of related paragraphs. Make sure you have composed complete paragraphs that present a point. The advice often given is that each paragraph should present one point only. Commence a new paragraph for each new point. Writing is a process, and you need to leave enough time to revise and edit your work from an initial draft, which may require further work to present ideas clearly and logically. Once you have your ideas on paper (based on your critical notes), reviewing your sentences, paragraphs and sections is more manageable. Similarly, in your presentations, you need to ensure that you use simple and straightforward language and logically structure your presentation so that your audience can follow your line of reasoning.

3. Use meta-commentary

You can help to lead or 'signpost' the reader or your audience through your written work or presentation by ensuring your ideas link together clearly. One technique is known as meta-commentary, where you begin by explaining how your assignment is structured, the topic and the essential ideas covered in the assignment. The Manchester Academic Phrase Bank gives helpful examples of how to introduce assignments and different sections of your work [https://www.phrasebank.manchester.ac.uk/].

4. Demonstrate your use of the best available information/ evidence

Select relevant and high-quality research, theory and policy for your presentation or writing. Demonstrate why you have chosen to refer to these resources. Remember to undertake a thorough search as outlined in Chapter 3. When you have a wide range of evidence, compare and contrast different authors' and researchers' perspectives when appropriate, then bring in your thoughts on these, linking to your own experiences in practice if appropriate.

Ensure the sources you refer to are relevant to your focus and the argument you are making. You will start this process when you search for information/evidence, but it is always worth reconsidering whether the information/evidence you use is the most appropriate for your case as you continue to write. Use the '**Six questions for critical thinking**' to help you to do this.

5. Use your own words rather than direct quotes from authors (avoiding plagiarism)

Using your own words to describe an author's work is much better than quoting directly from their work. When you cite a quotation, you do not demonstrate your understanding, whereas when you put the ideas into your own words (paraphrase), you show that you understand what the author intended. In other words, you should analyse and interpret (think critically about) what you have read rather than copy down or read out what other authors have said. The process involves breaking down their ideas/the meaning of what they are saying. In contrast, using many quotes in your work will suggest to your reader that you struggle to put what others have said into your own words. It may also suggest that you do not in fact understand what you have read, or that you find it hard to interpret it. Students often ask how to avoid the accusation of plagiarism – where you imply that the work of others is your own work. If you adhere to the principles above, you should avoid this charge.

6. Demonstrate your skills of critical appraisal and critical analysis

Give your reader or audience information about the types and quality of evidence you use. Information will help to show them that you understand and have thought carefully about the sources you are using, rather than just using the information/evidence that is most readily available. It also demonstrates that you are using the best evidence to support your academic work. You should avoid just citing a name and a date in your academic work with no further reference to the type of evidence you are referring to; otherwise, your reader or listener will not be able to tell if you are using the best available references. It is essential to use the right type(s) of evidence to back up your arguments – for example, if you are making a claim about how to manage a particular condition or situation effectively, citing research evidence will give you a much stronger case than if you cite someone's opinion. It would help if you then let your reader/listener know that your cited reference is research rather than opinion.

The following statements provide much more information than just citing the name of an author or researcher:

> - *An expert on this topic, Braemar (2023) suggests that …*
> - *As a result of a large-scale, high-quality systematic review, Jones et al. (2022) concluded that …*
> - *In this small qualitative study, Griffiths (2020) suggests …*
> - *In a multi-centred, international randomized controlled trial, Jacques et al. (2023) found that …*
> - *In this brief newspaper report on miscarriage rates in the UK in 2007, Davies (2023) speculated that …*
> - *Salkel (2023) bases her arguments and conclusions solely on her experiences of practice in hospitals as a student in the United States …*

When you incorporate critical appraisal of information/evidence into your writing, you can also point out any flaws or strengths in the arguments or ideas contained in what you have read, seen or heard, such as regarding the methodology of research studies, or the arguments of people you have spoken to. For example:

> *… although the study concludes that the treatment is effective, the small sample size and lack of inclusion of older people mean it cannot be applied to the general population.*

You will also demonstrate that you can think critically by comparing different authors' or researchers' views, and by noting when their arguments agree or disagree with each other. When you compose paragraphs, your critical thinking will be demonstrated through your evaluation sentences (see previous example). It would help if you analysed how strong their different arguments and conclusions are, linking this to your topic and your arguments. Again, use the '**Six questions for critical thinking**' to help you to do this.

7. Highlight alternative viewpoints

It is always valuable to highlight alternative viewpoints, thus demonstrating that you have looked at your topic from different perspectives. Addressing different viewpoints will be discussed further in Chapter 6. Where applicable and where possible, you should have a balanced view about the strength of the arguments you have considered.

8. Bring your points together (synthesize)

It is essential to bring your arguments together or 'synthesize'. Synthesis is the process of building up different ideas, evidence and pieces of information and then bringing them together into a coherent whole, to create new and original ideas and conclusions. Synthesis may include making recommendations for new approaches to practice (Cottrell 2011; Atkins and Schutz 2013). Synthesis also involves stating what you think overall, considering the issue or question as a whole, and weighing up the arguments and evidence you have analysed in detail. It is almost like taking a breath and saying, '*AND SO* …'. You may use similar words to those in your conclusion, but you also need to do this after considering each point or argument.

9. Summarize and conclude your work effectively

In your conclusion, you must bring together all the different synthesized points you have made; your conclusion should be clear, concise and based on the evidence you have presented. There should be no new information in the conclusion, which ideally should mirror what you set out to do in your introduction. Instead, you should sum up the key points you wish to highlight, and end with any recommendations for future practice and/or research. However, your conclusion may be tentative, in which case you will need to indicate this by using qualifying statements, phrases or words such as 'most', 'some', 'generally', 'it is possible that', 'in most cases', 'indicates', 'it would appear that', 'in a few cases', 'it is unlikely that', etc. Do not be afraid to state that no clear or convincing evidence exists for an issue. In fact, being tentative may demonstrate greater academic skill than coming to a strong conclusion for which you do not really have sufficient evidence.

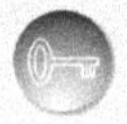

It is not enough to report what you see, hear or read. You must incorporate all the above strategies to demonstrate your critical thinking skills.

Review something you have written (e.g. an essay, assignment or report) or a presentation you have given. Do you think you demonstrated good critical thinking skills? How do you think you could have developed your work further?

Using different styles of writing and presenting

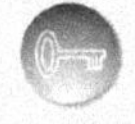

If you want to demonstrate critical thinking in your writing and presentations, you need to use the most appropriate writing or presentation style.

It is important to consider the types of writing styles you can use to demonstrate your critical thinking effectively within your written work. The main writing styles are:

- Description
- Explanation
- Evaluation
- Analysis
- Reflection.

Most good work that adopts a critical approach will incorporate all of the above writing styles. Some will, in addition, require a more personal *reflective* approach, which we discuss later in this chapter.

Description

Description is where information/evidence is given (verbally or in writing) in a factual manner. Description contains only information and facts – for example, saying what has happened, what something is like, what a theory says, or how something works. A description is helpful to set the scene with background information about a topic/issue or problem, a patient/client, a situation or an environment. Purely descriptive writing or presenting does not contain any explanation, evaluation, analysis or reflection, although the description may be the starting point for leading into these other writing styles.

The description should be concise. For example, when critically appraising a piece of research, it is important to briefly *describe the critical points* of the study before moving on to appraising and evaluating it. When reflecting on an event in practice, it is important to *describe it clearly and concisely first*, before you evaluate and analyse it in detail.

A description is essential in academic writing. It ensures that you tell the reader that you are familiar with the context and background of the ideas and the context in which you are working. However, in using only description, you would be *presenting and reporting* information/ideas, but *not developing them into your ideas or applying them to other contexts and thereby demonstrating your full understanding*. That is why description is often seen as a necessary component of academic writing but one that leads to writing where you can take a more critical approach.

Examples of descriptive language

- *Mrs Granta was a 56-year-old woman living alone in her one-bedroom flat. She had long-standing rheumatoid arthritis. She had been unemployed for six years and had been receiving benefits during this time. She was unable to walk far enough to reach her local shop, and relied on the support of her neighbour for shopping.*
- *Tang (2021) states that many university students regularly experience stress during their studies.*
- *Many carers of people with long-term conditions state that they experience feelings of frustration and isolation.*

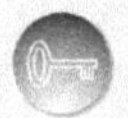

Introducing too much description into your writing or presenting will not give you the opportunity to incorporate evaluation, explanation, analysis or reflection. As a result, you will not have as much opportunity to demonstrate your skills of critical thinking.

Explanation

When using an explanatory style of writing or presenting, you provide *justification or reasons* for your ideas, views and arguments. **Explanation** is a step further than description as you provide additional information beyond the description. Explanation is used when you need to explain why an idea or concept is important, why you believe something, or why you have chosen to act in a certain way. Explaining may also involve giving further information about a word, phrase, focus or idea. For example, if given a broad topic area to explore, you may wish to explain why you have focused on certain issues.

You may be asked to provide a 'rationale' for your arguments and conclusions within your writing and presentations – this means that you need to give clear reasons and/or evidence to back up what you say. As a result, you will need to use words/phrases such as 'because', 'as' and 'due to' to back up your arguments.

Examples of an explanatory style (in bold font)

- *Travellers from non-endemic countries are at heightened risk of malaria **because they lack immunity** (WHO 2014).*
- ***Because Mr Khan did not have capacity to consent to his treatment and care,** I followed appropriate guidance from the Mental Capacity Act 2005 and ensured that we worked carefully as a team to act in his best interests.*
- *It was essential to use a non-confrontational and respectful approach when speaking to Mrs Oliver, **as I needed to minimize the tension and stress during our initial meeting**.*
- ***As Coddulph's small-scale quantitative study (2012) suggests that this intervention is ineffective,** I believe that a more extensive study should be carried out to confirm whether this is the case.*

Evaluation

Evaluation is about *judging and forming opinion, based on a sound argument* – this involves the *appraisal* of information or evidence. This style of writing is useful because it allows you to demonstrate skills in evaluating and appraising what you read, see or hear. This is important in all forms of writing and presentations, including essays, formal and informal reports, written and verbal reflections and presentations. For example, when evaluating research, you cannot simply say 'the research study was of high quality' – you also need to justify your comment by providing further information, and by referring to literature on research methodology. You should use the best available evidence to justify your views or conclusions.

The characteristics of and key points about evaluation in your writing and presentations are:

- You can demonstrate skills in weighing up the positive and negative aspects of an experience, concept or argument.
- You need to *justify* your view, giving a *reason* for your judgement – in other words, you need to combine evaluation with explanation (see above).
- Evaluation is likely to be combined with analysis and explanation, and it is also an essential part of reflection, which is discussed briefly below and in more depth in Chapter 5.

When evaluating information/evidence, refer to the '**Six questions for critical thinking**'.

Examples of an evaluative style (evaluative words in bold)

- *I feel that the strategies I used to establish rapport with Mrs Gonzales were **appropriate**, as she appeared to be relaxed during my visit, and she asked me if I could return to see her again – this, I feel, is an indicator of a **successful** first visit.*
- *While Barker et al. (2022) give a detailed account of their research methodology, and have a large sample size of participants, making their findings **more credible**, and their final conclusions are **fully justified**.*

Analysis

Analysis is about breaking down a topic, a concept, an issue, a question or an experience into parts. Instead of accepting the idea or concept at face value, analysis requires you to dig a bit deeper and look into the parts that make up the arguments. When analysing a topic, concept, issue, question or experience, you need to break down and explore in depth all the relevant information/evidence available to you.

The characteristics of and key points about analysis are:

- Analysis can offer a more objective, systematic and in-depth understanding of an issue.
- Analysis will come after description, evaluation and explanation.
- Analysis helps you to answer questions such as, 'What is going on here?', 'Why has this happened?' and 'What is this about?'
- If you use an analytical style of writing or presentation, you can compare different views or perspectives on a topic, issue or experience, and identify the differences between them. For example, in your writing or presentations, you may give two or three definitions of a key concept, referencing them. Then, by comparing and contrasting them, you can explain what is similar and what is different about the definitions.
- You can also show how different issues interrelate or influence each other.
- Analysis is a key part of critical appraisal and of reflection.

Example of an analytical style of language (analytical words in bold font)

*There are many, varied definitions of health. For example, Evans and Udal (2012: 15) focus **merely** on physical aspects, including 'the absence of disease'. **In contrast**, the World Health Organization (WHO 2006) **gives a more holistic perspective**, taking into account the physical, social, mental and spiritual aspects of a person's well-being. **Reflecting this**, in its Constitution, the WHO (2006) defines health as 'a state of complete physical, mental and social well-being and not merely the absence of disease or infirmity'.*

Good writing and presentation may include all of the components described above: description, evaluation, explanation and analysis in different measures depending on what is required.

Reflection

You may also need to use a reflective approach in your writing or presentations to explore your own and others' experiences and feelings about an event or issue being discussed. Reflective approaches to developing your practice are discussed further in Chapter 5. **Reflection** is about reviewing an experience in order to learn from it. Bulman et al. (2012) describe reflection as 'a process of searching for solutions to practice experiences, in order to make sense of them'.

The characteristics of and key points about reflection are:

- Using reflection can help you explore a complex issue in greater depth.
- Using reflection can help you to develop your self-awareness.
- By thinking critically and reflecting about an issue or event, you may be able to make more sense of it.
- If you write your reflections down, you are more likely to follow a structure.
- There are many reflective frameworks available (see Chapter 5). Most reflective frameworks involve description, analysis, evaluation, conclusions and planning, or a variety of prompts or questions to help you think in more depth about an issue.
- In addition to description, analysis and evaluation, you will need to explore your own and others' feelings and involvement in a situation or event.
- Reflection should involve creative thinking and may result in new understanding of an area or problem you are facing.

An example combining the above styles of writing

As stated above, you will most likely *combine* the above styles in your writing and presentations and, having done so, reach conclusions. In the simple extract below from a reflective essay or discussion (do note it is written in the first person, using 'I'), the different styles used are highlighted.

My appointment to visit Stephanie was scheduled at 10 a.m. (**description**). *We had agreed that this would be best, as her young daughter would be at nursery then* (**explanation**). *The aim of the visit was to explore Stephanie's feelings about fostering a child* (**description**).

Overall, although I was nervous (**feelings – part of reflection**), *I felt* (**feelings – part of reflection**) *that the visit was successful* (**evaluation**). *There are several reasons* (**explanation**) *why I have come to this conclusion. First, Stephanie said that she felt able to express her hopes, questions and concerns openly to me* (**explanation**). *This demonstrates that we had started to develop a therapeutic relationship, as described by Roberts (2013)* (**analysis**). *However, I do not believe that we had yet developed a true partnership. Secondly, I concluded that this visit partially met* (**evaluation**) *the local standards for good practice for home visits that my local authority (MCC 2021) has set out. However, we had not yet set goals as MCC (2021) indicates should be done on a first visit* (**analysis**). *Comparing this* (**analysis**) *visit to other similar visits that I have conducted in the past, I believe that this was one of the most satisfactory visits that I have ever conducted* (**evaluation**).

Students often ask about the use of first and third person – for example, whether they should say 'I searched the databases' or 'the databases were searched'. The answer is that both forms are acceptable. Unless your institution has a policy on the use of first or third person, you can use whichever form you prefer. Many journals request the use of first person as this can aid clarity in writing.

An example of applying critical thinking skills to written academic work

Imagine that a student called Michael has been asked to write a short academic report on the following topic:

> *Discuss the prevalence of smoking among pregnant women living in England, and analyse strategies currently used to reduce this, linking to relevant research, theory, policy and guidelines.*

Michael begins to research the topic area, and writes the first draft of his essay, which he shows to his tutor. An extract from this draft, along with his tutor's feedback, is shown below. Note how the tutor's comments link to the '**Six questions for critical thinking**' and to the language styles listed in this chapter. The superscript numbers in the extract refer to the tutor's comments below the extract.

Extract 1 – from Michael's first draft of his assignment

According to Action on Smoking and Health (2023),[1] just over 24 per cent of adults smoke. It is a well-known fact[2] that smoking in pregnancy is detrimental to the health of both pregnant women and their unborn children. Experts state[3] that smoking during pregnancy can cause miscarriage, stillbirth and underdeveloped babies, and can also increase the risk of cot death. According to Booth (2010),[4] children of women who smoke during pregnancy are also far more likely to be ill more often and are also much more likely to end up in hospital during the early stages of their lives.

It is essential, therefore, that all smokers who find themselves to be pregnant should be encouraged to quit smoking. According to Taniguchi et al. (2017),[5] there are many ways to give up smoking, for example using nicotine replacement therapy (NRT) via patches, gum, inhalators, lozenges or nasal sprays.[6] A variety of strategies can be used to deal with cravings, such as chewing gum, having a healthy drink or snack, or using some form of meditation, or focusing on the positive impact that giving up smoking will have on the foetus's health and development.[7]

Recent guidelines[8] state that women should be given a carbon monoxide breath test when they first book into maternity services, and should be asked if they smoke.[9] Women who say that they smoke should be referred to the NHS Stop Smoking Services, and should be given the telephone number of the NHS Pregnancy Smoking Helpline.[10]

There is much research on the effectiveness of different techniques to promote smoking cessation. Recent research suggests[11] that individualized approaches should be used in order to meet smokers' varying needs (Taniguchi et al. 2017).

This extract may at first glance appear to be well written and to incorporate a critical approach. The tutor's comments below, however, show how Michael's work could be developed further to enhance his critical skills within his writing.

Tutor's comments

1   What is this organization? Where did you find this information? You are quoting statistics from Scotland, related to the general population – could you 'dig deeper' to find a statistic more relevant to the focus of *pregnant mothers*, in *England*?

2   Who has stated this fact? You need to back up this statement with evidence – you need to demonstrate that you have carried out a systematic search for information and evidence related to your specific topic area.

3   Who has said this – which experts? You need to give references when you refer to others' work, and give more detailed information about your sources of evidence – remember the '**Six questions for critical thinking**'!

4   What type of evidence is this? **Like a newspaper report? It is an old reference**.

5   Who is this author, and where did you find this information? Is their work of good quality?

6   What exactly do the authors say about these different approaches in relation to pregnant mothers? Expand on this, introducing more analysis.

7   This is very descriptive. Do authors/researchers have any views about these? What are your own thoughts about these different options?

8   When were these guidelines written? Who has devised them, and how have they come up with these recommendations? You need to give a reference and explain their context in more detail.

9   What do you think of this approach? Have you had any experience of this strategy? If so, what are your thoughts?

10 Whose recommendation is this – is it your own? You need to be clear.

11 Is this research specifically related to smoking in pregnancy, or is it more general? You need to explain the context of these different pieces of research, and their methodology, analysing them in more depth, linking clearly to the focus of your assignment – *smoking cessation by pregnant women in England*.

Having read the above extract, and the tutor's comments, and bearing in mind what you have read so far in this chapter, write down how you think Michael could develop his work to demonstrate his skills of critical thinking more effectively in his writing.

There are a variety of ways in which Michael could enhance his work in order to demonstrate his skills of critical thinking more effectively in his writing. Here, we apply the principles of how to write critically and the 'top tips' we mentioned earlier in this chapter to this example.

To enhance his work, Michael could:

- **Plan his work more effectively before he starts** by using the '**Six questions for critical thinking**'.
- **Clearly identify the focus of his assignment.** Michael needs to start by analysing the assignment title/guidelines. He needs to note the key words within the title: for this assignment, he needs maintain his focus on *pregnant women who smoke in England*; and on discussing *strategies for promoting cessation* within this specific group of women. By doing this he will immediately demonstrate his skills of critical thinking, by showing that he can keep to this focus throughout his work.
- **Carry out an effective search for the best available evidence and information about his topic.** Michael needs to search for *relevant* and *high-quality* research, literature, statistics, policy and guidelines linking to his focus. He therefore needs to have skills in *searching effectively* and in *digging deeper* for relevant and high-quality information/evidence. He may need to contact a librarian for help with this.
- **Critically appraise the sources he finds as he researches the topic.** Michael then needs to *critically appraise* the information/evidence that he has identified in his search, *sifting* through all the information sources that he reads, sees and hears, such as research data, information from books, policy documents, and any information that he has been told in the practice setting. He could use the '**Six questions for critical thinking**' from Chapter 1 to help him identify the sources of information that are most relevant to his focus, and that provide the highest quality, authoritative evidence related to the topic.
- **Make critical notes throughout this process by using a systematic approach such as Cornell Notes.**
- **Compare and contrast different ideas/perspectives/research findings that he finds in the information/evidence he reads.** To enhance his work, Michael needs to demonstrate his ability to recognize and compare different viewpoints – for example, among authors, research findings and statistics – and to analyse and evaluate these

in a balanced way, where appropriate comparing them with his own experiences, ideas and views.

- **Back up statements with evidence.** Michael needs to ensure that any statements he makes in his work are backed up with good quality evidence such as research and high-quality sources of information/evidence that are clearly referenced.
- **Analyse the information/evidence he reads in greater depth.** Rather than just *reporting* information, Michael needs to *analyse it in more depth*, giving greater detail about what authors/researchers/reporters say, and discussing it in greater detail.
- **Ensure that his work is clearly and logically argued.** This will make it easier for the reader to understand Michael's ideas and follow his arguments.
- **Give a clear conclusion to sum up what he has learned.** Having considered the information/evidence he has read and linked it to his own experiences and observations, Michael needs to write a strong conclusion. It is important that he makes it clear how/whether his findings and conclusions will impact on his own and others' future practice – for further information on this, see the final section of the **'Six questions for critical thinking'**, **'So what?'**

Having taken his tutor's comments into account, Michael then works on a second draft of the assignment. He starts by ensuring that he is clear about what the assignment question is telling him to focus on; he then writes a plan or draws a spider diagram and finds authoritative, relevant information and evidence relevant to this topic. He takes time to write carefully in order to try to put his ideas across as clearly and logically as possible, demonstrating his skills of critical thinking.

What elements of effective critical writing that have been discussed in this chapter can you recognize in Michael's second draft of his work?

Extract 2 – from Michael's final draft of his assignment, demonstrating a higher level of critical thinking

In this assignment I will discuss the prevalence of smoking among pregnant women in England. I will then explore the strategies used to encourage pregnant women to give up smoking.[1] To set the scene, The

Information Centre (2022) stated that in 2020, 32 per cent of mothers who had recently given birth in England[2] said that they had smoked in the 12 months before or during pregnancy; 17 per cent of these mothers continued to smoke throughout their pregnancy. Younger mothers are more likely to smoke throughout pregnancy. These statistics indicate a continued need for action against maternal tobacco smoke exposure in order to eliminate harm to both the mother and the foetus that results from this.[3] However, these statistics should be read with a degree of caution, as smoking may be under-reported by pregnant mothers[4] (Taniguchi et al. 2017; NICE 2020). The reasons for potential under-reporting of smoking by pregnant mothers should be identified and considered carefully. By doing this it may be possible to encourage more pregnant women to be open about their smoking, so that they can be supported to quit.

There is growing evidence from epidemiological studies that smoking in pregnancy can be detrimental to the health of both pregnant women and their unborn children (NICE 2020). While the effects of smoking are not the focus of this report,[5] it is clear that those who run health and social services in England should see the promotion of smoking cessation in pregnant mothers, and in women contemplating getting pregnant, as a high priority.

There is evidence that a range of approaches can assist with smoking cessation. In a systematic review, Grange et al. (2020) identified that many types of non-pharmacological interventions had a moderate effect on smoking cessation and concluded that smoking cessation interventions in pregnancy are somewhat successful in reducing the proportion of women who continue to smoke in late pregnancy, and reduce the incidence of low birth weight and premature births. They concluded that health care professionals should be mobilized to employ a range of methods to reduce the incidence of smoking in pregnancy. Specifically, Taniguchi et al. (2017) undertook a cohort study of women who were receiving an intervention to assist smoking cessation.[6] Women were followed up in the study for 12 months, meaning that it was not clear whether the smoking cessation would continue beyond this point; although for the purposes of smoking within pregnancy this time span is sufficient. They found that the intervention was effective at reducing smoking, although details of the actual nature of the intervention were limited. In a smaller qualitative study, Stacey et al. (2022) explored the experiences of pregnant women who smoke in order to identify how smoking cessation services are received. They identified the need for a sympathetic and non-judgemental approach to women but acknowledged that their sample was small.[7,8]

In June 2020, the National Institute for Health and Care Excellence published official guidelines for assisting women to quit smoking during pregnancy and following childbirth. The guidelines are aimed at managers and professionals working in England and Wales in health care services, local authorities, education, and the private, voluntary and community sectors. The guidelines promote a sensitive, client-centred approach, acknowledging that some women may be reluctant to say that they smoke.

In summary,[9] it is clear that there is much effort taking place to reduce the incidence of smoking in pregnant women in England. Health and social care practitioners, myself included, will benefit from keeping up to date with developments in research and policy in relation to this aspect of their practice, in order to identify successful evidence-based strategies that may assist pregnant women to quit smoking.

Tutor's comments

- Good – you have clearly set out your focus at the beginning of your work, and set out your plans for how you will structure your report.
- Good – this statistic is specific to England, directly relevant to your focus. In a longer piece, you could expand further on this to compare different statistics.
- Good – you have set the scene for your work with relevant statistics.
- Well done – you have noted the potential limitations of the statistics you have cited, demonstrating the ability to critically appraise and critically analyse what you read.
- Good – you are ensuring that you keep your work relevant to the focus of the question you have been set.
- Again, you are demonstrating that you have identified research that is relevant to the question you have been set, you can recognize what this evidence is and that you have been able to understand the key conclusions from their research. Well done.
- This is relevant to your focus, which is good; but do you know where these papers came from? Were the papers all based on smoking cessation services in England?
- The conclusions you draw from this paper are tentative, which shows that you are able to distinguish between strong evidence and less decisive evidence. Well done.
- Good – you are summing up your work here.

Michael has now developed his work to demonstrate a more critical approach in his writing – he has ensured that his work is relevant to the question he has been set, and he has linked to relevant and high-quality sources of information/evidence, demonstrating that he has critically appraised them. As a result, his tutor's feedback is far more positive.

Michael's work could be developed further – this is just a small extract, but if he was able to write a longer piece, he could analyse the issues in even more depth, incorporating more critical analysis of a wider range of statistics, research and literature.

Demonstrating critical thinking in verbal presentations

We will now look at how you can demonstrate your skills of critical appraisal in your verbal presentations, and how you can prepare for delivering a presentation.

Many people struggle to demonstrate their skills of critical thinking and critical appraisal in their verbal presentations, and lack confidence in their abilities. It can be tempting to focus on *what content to include* in a presentation, rather than on *how the content should be delivered*, but both of these are important things to consider. It is easy to focus on just *presenting* or *describing* the information/evidence, rather than on explaining, evaluating, critically analysing or reflecting on it.

Many of the principles for incorporating critical thinking into your writing are also relevant to verbal presentations, and we covered these earlier in this chapter. It is worth revisiting them and thinking about how they might relate to presenting your ideas verbally.

Some 'top tips' for preparing and delivering a presentation

Before considering how to incorporate critical appraisal into your verbal presentations, here are some top tips you should consider when preparing to deliver one. These will help you develop confidence and competence when presenting.

- Check where your presentation will be delivered and at what time it is to start – can you access the venue in advance to set up?
- Check whether you have access to, and permission to use, audio-visual aids and other equipment – you may need to book it/bring your own.

- Check that you know how to use any equipment, so that you are not unduly nervous or distracted about using it – if you need help, find someone to show you.
- Rehearse! If possible, ask somebody to listen to you, to give you feedback on the content, pace and delivery of your presentation and to check your timings.
- Time yourself so you know how long it will take; be aware of any time limit you need to keep to, and don't overrun – part of the skill of being critical is being selective in what you say.
- Face the front, so that your audience can hear you, and speak clearly and slowly. Use notes rather than turn round to read your slides.
- Ensure you have some extra notes prepared in case you need to give additional information during or after the presentation.
- If you are using audio-visual aids, don't put too much information on each slide, and don't read off each slide word for word – this will make your presentation less interesting and less animated for the audience, and will not give you the opportunity to demonstrate your skills of critical thinking. Make sure the size of the print is large enough to be seen at the back of the room.
- Use a variety of approaches to break up your presentation (some questions, discussion, etc.).
- Consider letting your audience know in advance whether you will be giving out handouts/reference lists so that they don't have to take copious notes.
- If possible, you may wish to record your rehearsal and watch the recording yourself – this may help you to see how you need to develop your presentation skills.

Ensure you prepare for your presentation, rehearse and take into account the points made earlier in this chapter and the practical tips above. You should also bear in mind the following, to ensure that your skills of critical thinking are demonstrated clearly in your presentations.

- *Be clear about the focus of your presentation* and keep to this focus throughout – avoid becoming 'distracted' and discussing information and ideas that are not relevant to this.
- *Express yourself clearly, using simple terms* – do not assume that your audience will understand complex language and terminology, or abbreviations.

- *Link to relevant research, theory and policy,* demonstrating your skills of critical analysis and appraisal as you do so. Demonstrate that you have thought broadly about your topic and challenged your own assumptions and perspectives on the topic.

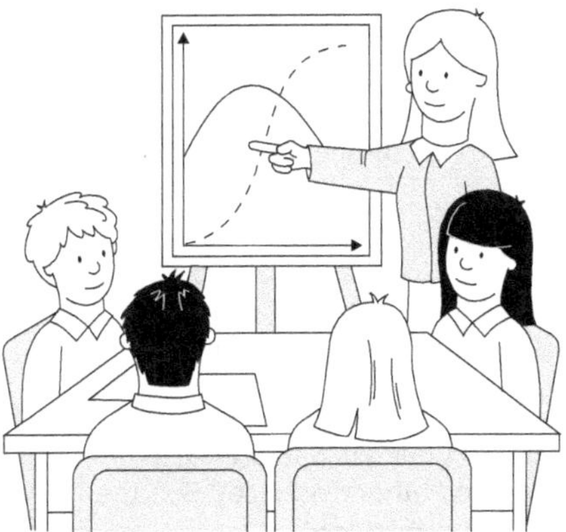

Figure 4.4

- Be prepared to *invite questions from the audience,* using them as an opportunity to demonstrate your skills of critical appraisal further. Be ready to link your answers/responses to relevant theory and research and ensure that you link the questions back to your focus.
- *Elaborate* on some of the points in your presentation – this is where you can use your critical thinking skills. For example, you can *evaluate* information/evidence, *analyse* a definition and *explain* complex terms.
- Ensure that *your argument is logical* and that *your conclusion is clear,* resulting from the process of synthesis.

A checklist for assessing your critical thinking in written work and presentations

It is important to apply the same rigour to your own writing and presenting as you do when analysing source materials. Below is a simple checklist to help you ensure you are demonstrating your skills of critical thinking in your writing and presentations. It can help you to see how you can develop your work further. You could also adapt this checklist and ask your peers to critically appraise your work and give you feedback – you may then get fresh ideas about how you can enhance your work.

A checklist for assessing your critical thinking in written work and presentations	Yes	No	Not sure
Have you composed critical notes to refer to?			
Have you set out clear aims?			
Have you explained your focus clearly to the reader/listener?			
Have you kept to this focus throughout your work?			
Have you selected sources of information/evidence that are relevant?			
Have you chosen high-quality sources of information/evidence and, where required, justified your choices?			
Have you demonstrated your skills of critical appraisal of research and other evidence? See the **'Six questions for critical thinking'**			
Have you put together a clear and logical argument, so that it is easy to follow your ideas?			
Do you need to revise sentences, paragraphs and sections to ensure that your reader is signposted?			
Have you demonstrated your ability to compare and contrast different authors'/researchers'/policymakers' perspectives in a balanced way?			
Have you put authors'/researchers' findings, ideas and perspectives into your own words, to demonstrate your understanding of their ideas?			
Have you appraised authors'/researchers' findings, ideas and perspectives in a balanced way, even when these contradict your own?			
Have you referenced all resources you have referred to in a systematic way in your text/presentation and in your reference list?			
Is your conclusion clear, and based on the evidence you refer to?			
Can you think of any ways that you could develop your work further? If so, note your ideas here:			

In summary

In this chapter, we have discussed why it is important to incorporate critical thinking into your writing and presentations. We have explained and introduced approaches to demonstrate critical thinking in your writing and presentations. We have also explored how you can plan your written work and presentations effectively. Finally, we have discussed how you can effectively present your critical thinking skills in your writing and verbal presentations. We have given some examples of critical writing for you to look at, to help you to develop your writing skills further. We have also provided some 'top tips' and a checklist to help you to plan your writing and your verbal presentations, and to help you demonstrate your ability to be critical in your work.

Key points

1   Incorporating a critical approach in your writing and presentations will demonstrate that you are well informed, and that you are able to identify relevant information/evidence and appraise the sources of information/evidence that you come across.
2   You will be more able to adopt a critical approach if you plan your work effectively before you start to write or put together your presentation.
3   Remember that planning includes undertaking a systematic search of the literature and being critical of what you find, using our '**Six questions for critical thinking**' (see Chapter 1) and enhanced by a method such as Cornell note-taking.
4   When citing a reference, try to give some information about the quality of the source and why it backs up the point you are making. Note the quality and type of source – for example, is it research or opinion based?
5   Ensure that your work is logically structured and well argued.
6   Seek feedback on your writing and your presentations from those around you, and critically appraise your own work to help you to develop it further.

5 Adopting critical thinking in your professional practice

- *The professional context and complexity of critical thinking – connecting theory and practice*
- *How you can think critically about the influences on your professional practice: routine, relying on your experience, using professional judgement and learning from others*
- *Assessing and developing your skills as a critical thinker*
- *Using questions to develop a more in-depth approach to critical thinking*
- *Influencing the 'critical thinking' culture of your workplace*
- *In summary*
- *Key points*

In this chapter, we will:

- Discuss the context and complexity of critical thinking in professional practice.
- Explore how you can think critically about routine, relying on your experience, using professional judgement and learning from others.

- Discuss how you can start to assess and develop skills for critical thinking in delivering safe and effective person-centred practice.
- Discuss how you can develop and use skills of reflection.
- Consider which aspects of your practice you do well and which aspects you may need to develop and how you can do this.
- Seek out evidence to inform your practice.
- Examine how you can use questions to develop a more in-depth approach to critical thinking.
- Offer top tips for influencing the 'critical thinking' culture of your workplace.

The professional context and complexity of critical thinking – connecting theory and practice

As discussed in Chapter 1, critical thinking is about having a curious, investigative and questioning attitude. Critical thinking involves having an approach to your professional practice that is thorough and analytical. These characteristics and approaches should be adopted in your practice incorporating where possible a critical approach to reading and appraising information/evidence.

In the health and social care professions, there is little point in being able to understand and critically appraise sources of information/evidence (see Chapters 2 and 3), or in being skilled at using critical thinking in your writing and presenting (see Chapter 4), if it makes no difference to the decisions you make and the management or care of your patients/clients. This is where theory and practice collide.

Similarly, there is no point having the sound qualities to be an excellent health or social care professional if you don't have the skills to think critically about information/evidence that underpins what you do. The idea that academic skills relate only to work within classrooms is unsafe and outdated. Aveyard, Greenway and Parsons (2023) discuss the multiple barriers to using evidence in professional practice and the reality that this is an ongoing issue that we need to continue to address. This might include developing an academic culture where research is valued within both the university and practice areas.

In environments that are often pressured and challenging, professionals need to adopt practical ways of incorporating a critical approach to practice into their everyday working lives. We offer some initial ideas for professionals and go on to suggest ways of developing further as a critical thinker.

We have argued in this book that we should deliver safe and person-centred care, as well as compassionate care. As outcomes and standards for health and social care are increasingly under scrutiny, it is important that as a student or qualified professional you adopt a critical thinking approach in your everyday practice. This will ensure you deliver safe and effective practice, as you will be fully considering what you do and why you do it. Standards that underpin health and social care practice are available widely and from all the countries of the UK (see useful web links section in this book). A major report by Francis (2013) in the UK, which is still very relevant today, has highlighted some deficiencies in standards of care, and noted how the organization in question had lost sight of the patient as it concentrated on targets to be met. To avoid such poor practice and organizational failings, professionals are more likely to meet high standards of health and social care by adopting a critical thinking approach. Indeed, to continue to develop personally and professionally, we need to strive to be critical thinkers.

See if there are quality standards for your own health and social care services and consider how, as a practitioner, thinking critically will help you meet such standards.

We referred to Price and Harrington's (2019: 13) detailed definition of critical thinking in Chapter 1. It is the latter part of their definition that connects more explicitly with professional practice. They say that critical thinking enables us to '*act as a knowledgeable doer – someone who selects, combines, judges and uses information in order to proceed in a professional manner*'. This is particularly pertinent as it asserts that we need to adopt the skills of critical thinking in order to practise professionally. The professional bodies in the UK make a clear connection with this in their standards of professional and ethical conduct. Other countries around the world may also have access to professional standards and policies that allude to some of these critical thinking attributes and skills.

What do the professional bodies say?

Access the standards or guidelines from your own professional body to see what they say about the need to be a critical thinker in professional practice.

In Chapter 1, we outlined that all health and social care professions are accountable for their practice. In addition, in the UK the Health and Care Professions Council (HCPC 2012) and the Nursing and Midwifery Council (NMC 2018) state in their codes of conduct that professionals need to ensure their practice is safe and effective. The HCPC (2012) adds that if you make informed, reasonable and professional judgements in the best interests of service users, you are likely to meet the standards of your profession. Here there is recognition that the judgement of professionals is an essential part of the care process. This involves critical thinking.

The NMC (2018) provides further guidance on this by stating that nurses and midwives should participate in appropriate learning and practice activities to maintain and develop their competence and performance.

Consider the following and jot down your initial thoughts:
If you are a student or a practice assessor/mentor, you may wish to consider whether there is an emphasis on critical thinking, evidence-based practice and accountability in the current pre-registration curriculum for your profession. You can usually establish this from your professional body website. If you qualified a while ago, you may wish to see how this emphasis has changed over time. As a qualified professional, you will not be able to maintain your professional knowledge and status by relying on your initial pre-registration education – you will need to consider a 'lifelong learning' and 'continuous professional development' (CPD) approach. In order to do this, we now consider how you can think critically about *routine, your own experience* and *learning from others.*

How you can think critically about the influences on your professional practice: routine, relying on your experience, using professional judgement and learning from others

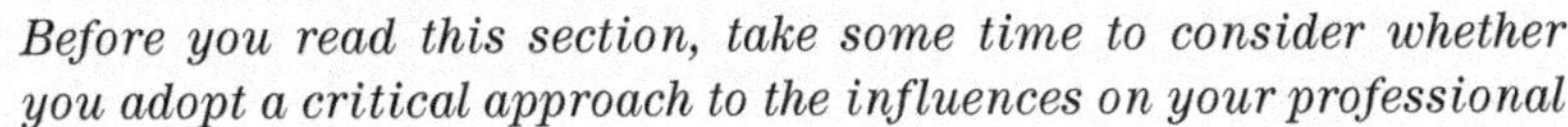

Before you read this section, take some time to consider whether you adopt a critical approach to the influences on your professional

practice. For example, do you think critically about and reflect on your role in delivering safe, effective and compassionate care, or do you just follow routines and/or rely on your own or others' experiences?

Thinking critically about routine

In our busy day-to-day working lives (as students or professionals), it is sometimes practical to adopt the practices that are used by those more experienced than us. This is, of course, useful when we have little or no knowledge or skill ourselves, or need to act quickly or want to fit into a working environment. However, when we think critically, we shouldn't just carry on adopting these approaches without question and do things *the way they have always been done.*

Using the following table we have developed, think about some recent working days/practice shifts and **assess on the scale between 5 and 1** *to what extent you feel you demonstrate a critical attitude/approach to your practice.*

If in the main you scored yourself towards the left, with high scores, then you are probably *thinking critically* about your practice. If you tended towards scoring yourself towards the right-hand statements, then you may be adopting more routinized – and therefore less critical – approaches to your practice. In either case, you may wish to consider how you might further develop a critical approach by reading the 'top tips' later in this chapter.

Approaches to practice: 'critical thinking' or relying on routine

◄——————Identify where your practice lies ——————►
on a scale of 5 to 1

I do this	5	4	3	2	1	I do this
I often challenge the routine and try to be flexible in how I work to meet the needs of my clients						I do as I am told to do and keep to the routine
I am proactive in seeking out new practices						I do as I have been taught in the past
I see my work as a profession with responsibilities						I see my work as a job
I am able to confidently question the ideas/ practices of others						I would not feel confident questioning the ideas or practices of others
I welcome constructive challenge of my practice						I would be upset or angry if someone questioned what I did
I proactively seek out and take up opportunities to attend a wide range of development activities						I only attend essential training and development, even when other opportunities for development are available to me
I have read a variety of research and/or new policy in the last 12 months						I have not read research or new policy in the last 12 months
I feel confident explaining the reasons for my decisions						I avoid offering more than basic explanations for my decisions

(continued)

I often look up new knowledge in books, journals or professional online resources						I rarely access a book, journal or professional online resource
I often reflect on my day/shift						I forget about work once I have finished my day/shift
I regularly ask colleagues for feedback on my practice						I rarely ask for feedback on my practice

Spot what you and others say. Highlight which of the quotes below might indicate a critical approach to practice versus a routine and unquestioning approach:

'I often wonder why we do things a certain way.'
'I am interested in what is going on in the world.'
'This is how we do it here.'
'We have always done it like this.'
'If I spot inconsistencies, I ask why?'
'In my experience …'
'I read recently that there is a new approach to …'
'I do the same as my colleagues, so it must be all right.'
'We often discuss what the best practice is, and someone usually offers to find out more if need be.'
'No one has complained.'
'I regularly look things up on the internet if I am not sure.'
'I heard about it at a conference/seminar.'
'It is in the guidelines/policy/standards.'
'I don't really have a say in how it's done.'
'I asked my student and he told me this is how they are taught.'
'A practice assessor/mentor told me this is how they do it!'
'I've got a really "difficult" student who asks questions all the time.'
'We can't use the best … we don't have the money for it.'

There is no right answer for each of the quotes above, and for many we could say that 'it all depends'. If we have considered things critically, then our practice should be safe and effective. For example, 'doing the same as colleagues' may indeed be best practice, *if you have questioned* what informed their practice. It is fine to 'follow policy and guidelines' *if you have thought critically* about how up to date and relevant they are. However, if you just do as someone tells you to do without question, then you would *not be thinking critically*. For example, imagine the following scenario:

Scenario: Mark

Mark (a health or social care professional) is confident and comfortable in his role. He works hard, is well liked and responds to requests for help from colleagues. He arrives at work and is clear about what needs to be done. However, he sometimes struggles to respond to students' queries about the reasons for certain interventions.

He then decides to apply for funding to go to a conference. He meets other professionals in similar roles to his own. He discusses his working practices and, through sharing ideas, discovers that several interventions or approaches he has been using are out of date. Mark comes to realize that these may have been delaying the recovery or support of his patients/clients. It was only through discussion with colleagues and by finding new information that he was able to challenge his approach to his work and become more critical about his practice. He came back to work energized and motivated to keep learning and to learn from, and with, his future students.

People who think critically are aware that there is a lot to learn, that they don't know everything and that they are on a professional journey. Being comfortable in your work may indicate that you are settled into a routine and adopting a ritualistic approach.

Some benefits of routine working

- It provides structure to your day.
- You may feel comfortable and in control, knowing what to expect.
- It can improve efficiency of tasks.
- You and your colleagues can work out time-frames and know what to expect from each other.
- When new members join a team, it can make it easier for them to 'pick up' what needs to be done, where and how.

Wolf (2014) discusses the importance of rituals in nursing and says that nursing owns its rituals in the same way that it has a culture.

He explores how some cultural groups have rituals to develop their identity and social interactions. Carrying out ritualistic practice can be a response to anxiety, as it is often comforting to do the familiar. However, in the context of practice development, McCormack et al. (2013) suggest that there has been a shift away from ritual and routine as health and social care professionals embrace the more individual and context-based approaches to care.

Negative things about routine working

There are also some negative aspects of continuing with routine working and ignoring or failing to access new evidence. Greenway (2014) discusses rituals in nursing and specifically intramuscular injections. Despite the fact that the evidence suggests a particular site for such injections, she notes that practitioners are reluctant to change and they continue to adopt familiar and dated practices.

If you always do things the same way:

- You may not develop new and creative approaches to your practice.
- You may not meet the individual needs of your patients/clients.
- Your work may be boring and predictable and you may not get job satisfaction.
- When the unexpected happens, you may not be able to adapt.
- You may not be able to cope well with fluctuating workloads.

Example: A change in routine ...

A patient/client is confused and aggressive and is disturbing others. The approach most often used to deal with such a situation is to call security or sedate the client. Many staff assume that these are the only ways to deal with aggression. A new member of staff who has worked in other settings suggests adopting a more person-centred approach, and says they have used distraction as a successful approach in similar situations in the past. She has applied her personal knowledge, challenged the assumptions of the accepted practice and tried an alternative technique to try to meet this patient's/client's interests. This shows a critical thinking approach.

Rather than concluding that there is only one way to deal with a situation, it is better to be open to, and actively seek, alternatives. This requires critical thinking.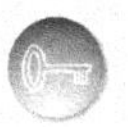

Thinking critically about experience

You may be an experienced practitioner or even a final-year student and feel that what you have learned from your past experience enables you to function at a more advanced level in your professional role. The development from novice to expert has been discussed widely in both education and practice since Patricia Benner wrote her book, *From Novice to Expert*, in 1984. On its own, experience is not enough to guide practice; however, there is implicit agreement that the development of experience and intuition is a hugely valuable resource (Sicora et al. 2021). The contribution that experience makes to our professional practice is very hard to quantify and equally hard to research. In a cross-sectional study, Lang et al. (2013) found there was no significant association between critical thinking skills and years of experience.

We would therefore argue that safe and effective practice is achieved not only by relying on experience, but also developing skill in making effective judgements and decisions using evidence. Just as you need to be critical of the information/evidence you have, you also need to be critical of using your own experience to guide practice. Thinking back to the definition of evidence-based practice given in Chapter 1, you will remember that using evidence, professional judgement and patient/client preference contributes to an evidence-based approach.

__Experience alone is not enough.__ Our __professional judgement__ is likely to be most effective when it is based on the best available information/evidence so that we can consider a wide range of __alternatives__, __assumptions__ and include the __perspective of patients/clients__.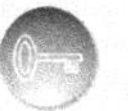

Defining professional judgement

Thompson et al. (2013: 1721) simplify the notion of making judgements as 'the assessment of alternatives'. They give 'is this patient/ client deteriorating or not?' as an example of when you might need to make an evaluation. This assessment of alternatives will usually need to be followed by the making of a decision as to which direction to take. A critical thinker will be open to a wider range of alternatives and question their own and others' assumptions and so is therefore more likely to make sound judgements and decisions.

Standing (2011: 7) defines professional judgement as:

Informed opinion (using intuition, reflection and critical thinking) that relates observation and assessment ... to identifying and evaluating alternative ... options.

In health and social care practice, there are many instances of uncertainty and so there are likely to be many opportunities to use our professional judgement. As Standing (2011) notes, this includes critical thinking and reflection. We will discuss reflection later in this chapter.

Thinking critically about learning from others

When you don't have much experience yourself (maybe as a student or as a qualified professional in a new environment), you may learn by working alongside others. However, even when you are working with experienced and respected colleagues or practice assessors/mentors, you need to think critically about *how* you use them as role models. Over the years, there has been much written about 'role modelling'. Bandura (1965) described how individuals tend to adopt the practices demonstrated by those they hold in high regard. This approach to learning may be useful in some situations, such as when learning complex skills or behaviours. Baldwin et al. (2014) report that there is some research on role modelling in medicine and nursing but little in other professions, although most professionals can recall someone who they looked up to, respected and wanted to emulate. Jochemsen-van der Leeuw et al. (2013) carried out a systematic review of role modelling in clinical teachers and found that many of the characteristics of both positive and negative role models came under the categories of patient/client care qualities, teaching qualities, and personal qualities. For example, a positive role model displays professional behaviours and is supportive, whereas negative role models can be unfair or cynical.

You may use role models for your professional practice, or you may be able to select a role model for critical thinking. Lovatt (2014) explores, summarizes and applies to professional education the work of Brookfield (2012), who argued that educators could be role models for critical thinking by using personal examples of how they have sought out and checked assumptions and demonstrated that they can be critical thinkers themselves. The other way educators can model critical thinking is by being clear about the purpose of activities or assignments – so that learners are clear about what is expected of them. Felstead (2013) adds that if learners can see educators demonstrating their thought patterns, they are more likely to model that behaviour. So as well as modelling safe, effective and compassionate practice, professional educators can model their thinking too.

Positive role models possess professional competence, critical thinking skills and personal qualities that you may want to adopt. But you should think critically about the credibility of the role models themselves. If you are a role model to others, you should think critically about how you may be seen, both positively and negatively. 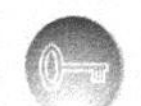

By reflecting on this, you may become more self-aware of how you come across to others as a role model. Although you may learn excellent approaches to your professional practice from others, it is not good practice to accept/emulate others' practice without question, as their approach may not be the most suitable. As professionals or students, we should be aware of the potential danger of modelling from, or being a role model for, negative attributes.

Try to identify someone in an education setting or in professional practice who is a critical thinker. What qualities and behaviours do they demonstrate that you can emulate? 

You may also be a role model yourself to others now or in the future. This makes it even more important to adopt a critical thinking approach to your professional practice.

'Top tips' for thinking critically when learning from others

If you are seeking advice from colleagues or practice assessors/ mentors about an issue in practice, you may want to consider using all '**Six questions for critical thinking**', but specifically the ones highlighted here.

> **Question 3** asks: **Who has said this?** You should consider if the person you are learning from:
>
> - Has expertise? *How do they keep up to date? Can they give a clear rationale for their advice? What qualifications do they have?*
> - Is trustworthy? *Do they have any reason (pride, own agenda, embarrassment, concern about status, etc.) to 'bluff' or give you false information or advice? Consider if they readily admit to being wrong or are open to challenge.*
> - Models a critical thinking approach?
> - Is reflective?
> - Seeks out and challenges assumptions?
>
> Regarding the information/evidence they are giving you, **Question 1** asks, **What is it?**, while **Question 6** asks, **How do you know it is good quality?** You should consider the following:
>
> - How full and detailed is the information/evidence they have provided? *Do you have the full picture? Where does the information/evidence come from?* Request the source of the information they are giving you (e.g. policy, guidelines, research, review) and look at it yourself.
> - What are the risks or consequences involved in accepting or rejecting their advice? *Can you check it out from other sources? Are there any policies, guidelines or research evidence to help in the decision-making?*

We have explored how relying on routine, experience and learning from others without question can lead to an uncritical approach. You are likely to be thinking critically if you question and consider fully all aspects of your practice, including when you might be adopting routines, rituals or the advice or experience of role models. We will now consider further how you can think more critically about your professional practice and explore what you can do as an individual to develop a critical approach in your day-to-day practice.

Assessing and developing your skills as a critical thinker

Self-assessment tools

Facione (2013: 13) offers a 'critical thinking disposition self-rating form' that can help you determine whether you have a positive or adverse approach to critical thinking based on your actions in the previous few days. Paul and Elder (2014) also offer a variety of tools to develop yourself as a critical thinker and say it needs to be practised to be fully developed (although their writing does not relate specifically to health and social care). Many employers in industry use critical thinking tools such as that of Watson and Glaser (2012), which tests for ability to recognize the skills of inference, assumption, deduction, interpretation and evaluation. See our useful websites appendix for links to download tests/tools.

Beginning to think critically

Once you have assessed your critical thinking abilities, we suggest three ways that you can start (or further develop) how you think about your professional practice in a more critical way:

1. Develop and use skills of reflection.
2. Consider which aspects of your practice you do well and which aspects you may need to develop and how you can do this.
3. Seek evidence to inform your practice.

Developing and using skills of reflection

Facione (2013: 16) describes how critical thinking is 'purposeful, reflective judgement that is focused on deciding what to believe or what to do'. Reflection is something that can be done by an individual or a group of individuals. Facione asserts that if we are being reflective and balanced in our views, we are using our critical thinking skills. However, it is not enough to have critical thinking skills; we also need the disposition or temperament to become a critical thinker. Critical thinking and reflection don't just happen – you need to be motivated and determined to make the best judgements you can. Barnett (1997: 1) advocates the development of 'critical being', which includes the development of self. He argues that, 'Critical persons are more than just critical thinkers. They are able critically to engage with the world and with themselves as well as with knowledge' (ibid.). We would argue that the skills of critical thinking are needed to reflect, and the skills of reflection are needed for critical thinking! Therefore, if we adopt a critical approach to reviewing our experiences, then this should enhance our learning and practice. Reflection requires us to demonstrate several of the same skills and qualities needed for critical thinking, including self-awareness, the ability to evaluate and analyse (Atkins and Schutz 2013).

Mann et al. (2009: 597) carried out a systematic review of reflection and comment that several definitions of reflection from the earliest to the more recent 'emphasise purposeful critical analysis of experience and knowledge in order to achieve deeper meaning and understanding'. This is because definitions of reflection and of critical thinking generally incorporate active mental processes (considering, reviewing, thinking) that involve some breaking down or analysis of the evidence or experience within a particular context and then reaching a conclusion or outcome.

Defining reflection

There are many definitions of reflection but they tend to encompass such things as considering feelings, experiences and moving towards a change or action (Bulman 2013a). The one below is useful in that it captures the practical nature of learning from reflection.

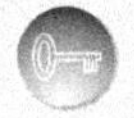

Reflection is a complex, widely defined and interpreted concept but, simply put, it is an approach to reviewing an experience in order to learn from it (Reid 1993: 305).

In their qualitative study exploring the concept of reflection from the perspective of both student and teacher, Bulman et al. (2012: e12) explain how:

> *Reflection was seen as a process of searching for solutions to practice experiences, in order to make sense of them. Student and teacher perceptions of reflection included the critical analysis of feelings and knowledge in order to lead to new perspectives about practice. Ultimately, reflection was connected with a professional motivation to 'move on' and 'do better' within practice in order to learn from experience and critically examine 'self'.*

Hargreaves and Page (2013) add that for health and social care professionals, intuitive and self-reflective behaviour is assumed and so there is an emphasis on deep personal and critical reflection.

There are many excellent texts and journal articles on reflection, and for a more in-depth insight it is suggested you read more widely (see, for example, Bulman and Schutz 2013; Jasper 2013). There is also a resource that has been written specifically for students (Clarke 2024). Clarke develops the definition of reflection by suggesting that it is about '*the empowerment of self through the understanding of self*' (2024:1). Reflective writing is discussed briefly in Chapter 4. In this chapter, we discuss further the types of reflective writing you may find useful specifically for your practice development. Although we are unable to discuss all aspects of reflection in this book, we suggest you consider the following areas to facilitate and incorporate reflection into your everyday professional life. It is a good idea to check out your self-awareness.

Developing and assessing your self-awareness

One of the skills or attributes of reflection is self-awareness. According to Goleman et al. (2013: 40), self-awareness involves 'having a deep understanding of one's emotions, one's strengths and limitations as well as one's values and motives'. And Atkins and Schutz (2013: 28) state that being 'self-aware involves being conscious of one's character, including beliefs, values, qualities, strengths and limitations'.

You probably think you have a good understanding of your personal strengths, qualities and skills and perhaps think you are aware of your limitations or weaknesses, but how do you know if your self-assessment is accurate? Part of critical thinking is to consider your own performance critically too. Goleman et al. (2013) note that a telling, but not always visible, sign of self-awareness is the ability to be reflective and thoughtful.

To check the accuracy of your own self-awareness, you could assess your own skills, knowledge, qualities, strengths and limitations in relation to an issue and then ask others for their perspectives. This will help identify whether your perspective is the same or different from that of others. If many other people see a situation differently or see your qualities and skills very differently from how you see yourself, you may want to question your self-awareness more closely. Most professionals have an annual appraisal or performance review, and this can help check out if our own self-assessment of our job performance is accurate. Students are often encouraged to self-assess before receiving feedback on a placement and this can achieve the same purpose when compared against the feedback. You may also be asked to be involved in 360-degree appraisal. This is where you are asked to make a self-assessment, which is then compared to the opinion of others such as peers, managers and subordinates.

Invite feedback on your strengths and areas for development from those you work with – those more senior to yourself, peers and/or more junior colleagues, as they will all offer different perspectives. If you are a student, work with different members of staff and see if they identify similar or different areas of strength and areas that you can develop further.

Using reflective frameworks

There are a variety of reflective frameworks available (e.g. Driscoll 2007; Johns 2010; and Gibbs 1988, which has now been adapted and updated by Bulman 2013b). Most incorporate an element of evaluation and analysis and so, as we have indicated throughout this book, using these approaches will ensure you are being critical in your day-to-day practice. Driscoll's (2007) 'What?' model of structured reflection, shown below (Figure 5.1), is a tool you can use easily in practice to enhance your critical thinking skills (see Chapter 4 for more ideas on description, analysis, evaluation and explanation). You can use reflective frameworks or models individually or with others, privately, or in some cases you may want to share your reflections.

It might be argued that the use of frameworks may be restrictive and that a free, less structured approach to reflection may be more creative. It may be worth trying different approaches to see what works for you.

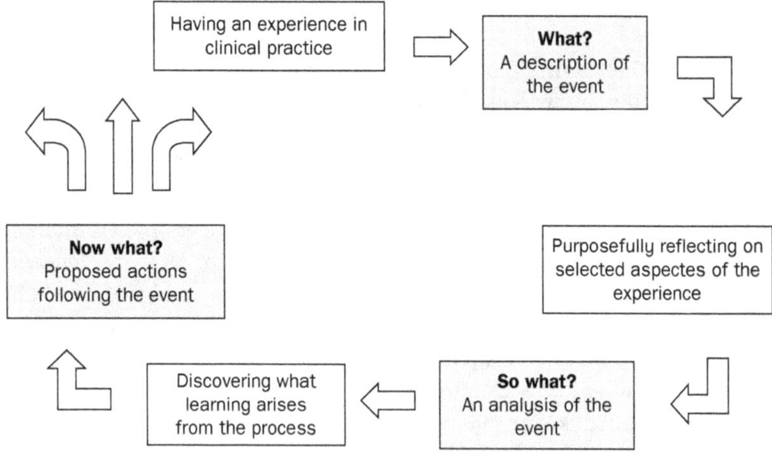

Figure 5.1 Driscoll's (2007) 'What?' model of structured reflection

Mann et al. (2009) reviewed 29 studies on reflection and found there was a lack of research on the outcomes of reflection. The authors also found, however, that reflection appears to make the meaning of complex situations clearer and so enables learning from experience. In other words, reflection helps you to be critical. You may want to consider how you can adopt a more reflective approach to your practice in a conscious and proactive way. We offer some suggestions below.

Keeping a reflective diary or learning journal

This may help you work through and learn from issues from your professional working life, and by being aware of the components of a reflective framework (in any order) you are more likely to incorporate a questioning approach that will ensure you are being critical. You may find that writing reflective accounts, even brief ones, can help you see things a little differently as you commit your thoughts and ideas to text. Once familiar with the components of structured reflection, you may find that you don't need to use a framework and can just write freestyle. Tate (2013) says that writing a personal journal should be about the journey or process rather than the outcome, and each individual needs to find out what works best for them. If you want to expand your writing, Johns (2010) offers a framework that moves you from just recording your experiences to examining them in more depth, including reflecting with others.

Keep a reflective diary for a few days. Use a structured approach and see if it impacts on the way you think about your practice. 

You could also identify a 'critical friend' or engage in 'professional/ clinical supervision' in order to gain more structured support for your reflection. Sometimes a more formal arrangement exists in the form of professional supervision and this can be with one other person or within a group, such as an action learning set. These approaches are now discussed in a little more detail.

Finding a 'critical friend'

A critical friend can help you as a professional or a student to make sense of a situation by commenting on and questioning your reflections. Bulman (2013b) notes that a reflective colleague can help open

Possible diary structure	
Initial reflection	**Additional thoughts/reading**
Example 1 *Today I saw a colleague move a patient/client without using a slide sheet. The patient looked uncomfortable and I was concerned for my colleague's own safety.* *I have had my own training on moving and handling and know that a slide sheet should be used. I didn't feel able to say anything as I was busy and didn't feel confident in how to challenge her …*	*Consider how I might challenge the practice of colleagues – maybe discuss in the department meeting so we all agree that we will do it?? Read more about local policy and guidelines.*
Example 2 *I was visiting a family in their home; the mother appeared reserved and nervous. Her husband tended to answer the questions I had and he didn't leave the room at all. I just felt something was wrong and couldn't say why. I noticed bruising on her lower arm, even though she had tried to cover it up. I felt I needed a way of offering her an opportunity to talk …*	*I need to explore family risk factors in more detail and make sure I am aware of the safeguarding policies and procedures. We could discuss as a team how to get information to clients who are vulnerable.*

up different perspectives, act as a sounding board, provide support and guide you. This requires a relationship of trust, honesty and openness. You will enhance your critical thinking by having your assumptions challenged and widening the perspectives you have.

Taking part in professional/clinical supervision or person-centred development

Bond and Holland (2010: 15) explain that clinical supervision is used to facilitate 'in-depth reflection on complex issues … this reflection is facilitated by one or more experienced colleagues'.

Professional/clinical supervision has been seen as a way of promoting personal development and regular reflection, usually between two people focusing on learning (Elliott 2013). There is an expanding evidence base for the practice of supervision (Catling et al. 2024). You may want to identify someone to discuss your practice with whose view you respect. If two or more professionals explore their thinking together, it can broaden perspectives, challenge assumptions and encourage questioning. Supervision can be achieved by meeting to discuss professional and practice issues in a non-threatening, supportive environment. The development of a trusting relationship is crucial. This can help produce a critical approach to professional practice in the following ways:

- By 'challenging' in a supportive way.
- By acting as a sounding board (so you can offer creative ideas and thoughts).
- By asking probing questions.
- By listening to each other's perspectives.
- By offering an expert opinion on a situation.
- By considering alternative options for solving an issue/problem.
- By using the '**Six questions for critical thinking**'.
- By giving time and attention to exploring significant professional issues.
- By acknowledging the emotional impact of challenging professional situations.

Taking part in 'action learning sets'

Action learning sets are one way of organizing group-based reflective learning. From our experience, it can be useful to reflect and discuss in groups when there is a particular common focus or area of interest. Dunphy et al. (2010a) describe how when action learning was used as part of a course, participants were able to discuss real problems that concerned them, although they did note some problems regarding participants' commitment to working in action learning sets. Carter (2013) describes how with group reflection there are benefits, such as learning from others; risks, such as individuals feeling anxious; and challenges, such as finding protected time.

Undertaking 'critical incident analysis' or debriefing

According to Vachon and LeBlanc (2011: 894), 'Critical incident analysis (CIA) is one of the strategies frequently used to facilitate reflective learning. It involves the thorough description and analysis of an authentic and experienced event within its specific context.' The analysis of personally significant (or 'critical') situations can be valuable in terms of identifying reasons why we act in certain ways or make certain decisions, in order to learn from those situations. The **critical incident technique** has been around for many years and Flanagan (1954) described how it was used to learn from the success or failures of pilots in flight training schools. It has been widely used in many professions, as a tool in education (Tripp 2011) and in health care and social work practice to aid critical reflection. It can help practitioners to uncover why they may have acted in a certain way and what has influenced their decision-making. It is also used as a research approach (see Hosie et al. 2014).

Debriefing is used after stressful or unusual events, in particular to learn from them. For example, Keene et al. (2010) discuss bereavement debriefing where professionals use a clear structure to explore specific cases. This involves exploring coping strategies and lessons learned using a series of prompt questions. Debriefing is often used following traumatic or unusual events.

Even a simple prompt such as 'tell me about it' can help a professional or student to discuss an issue, an incident or practice situation in their own way. Further prompt questions can be used once the reflection starts, as Brotherton and Parker (2008) suggest:

- What was the context?
- How were you feeling before or after the event or issue?
- What were you thinking?
- How did others see the event or issue?
- What were the consequences?

Developing your reflection further

There is much written about reflection and we recommend Bulman and Schutz (2013) for a more in-depth exploration. We would strongly assert that by adopting such reflective approaches, you will be thinking more critically about your professional practice. All of these reflective approaches are enhanced if you incorporate sound evidence at the analysis stage.

Consider which aspects of your practice you may need to develop

To identify which aspects of your professional practice you may need to develop, you can start by purposefully and critically thinking about, or reflecting on, all aspects of your own work – this means adopting a questioning approach to all that you read, see, hear and do in relation to your practice. To ensure this you could:

- Imagine you are new to a job (or as a student/learner new to a placement). What would your impressions be and would you see anything that you might consider to be unprofessional, unjustified or routine?
- Use team discussions and observations to identify which areas of practice you and your colleagues approach in an uncertain or inconsistent way.
- Consider and reflect upon what the reasons are for the way you carry out your practice and then consider how you can move to a more critical and evidence-based approach.
- Reflect on the management of a patient/client to see how you could improve this.
- Consider any feedback you have from patients/clients and how person-centred your approach to care is.
- Undertake a SWOT analysis (explained below).

In Chapter 1, we introduced the term 'critical analysis' and explained how it involves breaking down a situation or the written word. Although the origin of the SWOT analysis tool is unknown and there are some that criticize its theoretical underpinnings, it is often used as an evaluation and planning tool in business, the professions and education (Helms and Nixon 2010). We have found it to be a useful tool for exploring professional practice. It provides a simple framework for you to consider an issue or an aspect of practice.

Undertake a SWOT analysis (see below) of a particular aspect of your practice within your workplace. You could look at any of the following: 

communication with patients/clients; team working; documentation; patient/client experiences of care; or management of a particular patient/ client intervention or problem. The Mindtools website offers some helpful explanations of doing a personal SWOT analysis or a professional one of your work environment [http://www.mindtools.com/pages/article/ newTMC_05.htm]

SWOT analysis tool	
Strengths	Weaknesses
Opportunities	Threats

Seeking out and exploring the evidence for your practice

In Chapters 2 and 3, we explored different types of information/evidence and distinguished between 'readily available' and 'best available' evidence. If you wish to develop as a critical thinker in practice, you need to be questioning and strive to find the best available evidence for your interventions. It isn't possible to suddenly be able to give solid evidence-based reasons for everything (big and small) that you do on a daily basis, and so it may be better to start with some small changes. Being a critical thinker involves you being thoughtful and questioning about information/evidence but also discussing your practices with your colleagues.

Think more critically about your professional knowledge base – use any of the following ideas to make even a small change in the way you think critically about the information/evidence you use in practice:

- Ask 'WHY?' more often!
- Use our '**Six questions for critical thinking**'.
- Get training in using professional databases to search for evidence.
- Look initially to see if there are any systematic reviews that are relevant [for example, see https://www.cochrane.org/cochrane-reviews *or* https://www.campbellcollaboration.org/].
- See if your workplace or placement area has a library or offers online access to resources.
- Start practising systematic searching for just one or two important issues as discussed in Chapter 3. This is so that you access the 'best

available' information/evidence rather than relying on what comes most easily to hand.

- Determine whether there are any national guidelines on key areas of your professional practice. For example, in the UK: 'Evidence and best practice resources', available to everyone in health and social care [see https://www.nice.org.uk/about/what-we-do/evidence-services].
- Look one thing up every day. Try to use professional and good quality sources of information/evidence.
- Visit other similar specialties or areas, and network with colleagues who do similar jobs (at conferences and training sessions or informally). This will enable you to 'check out' what is considered best practice.
- Be open to the fact that *'you may not know what you don't know'*. Exposure to other people, education and organizations may help ensure you are not missing out on key knowledge or perspectives.
- Set up a journal club. Such clubs can be useful to inform professionals and embed evidence-based practice and are increasingly using social media as a platform (Leung et al. 2013).
- Reflect on your practice regularly.
- Ask experts or students to share their knowledge with your team through teaching sessions or presentations (remember to think critically about what they say!).
- Identify study days, courses and conferences relevant to your practice and ask for study leave and/or funding to attend.
- Follow the news for health or social care stories that widen your perspective.
- Ensure that individuals who attend any development opportunities feed back to the whole team.

If possible, use a professional database and search systematically for evidence for your practice as discussed in Chapter 3. 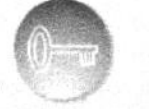

Positive approaches to questioning/challenging practice

We are likely to be part of small and local or larger teams when working in health and social care. There are ways in which you can use these teams to ask questions, share ideas and practices. You could discuss with colleagues how you might develop a 'questioning culture'. This is where everyone considers it positive to ask each other why certain approaches are adopted. If you are taking a critical thinking approach yourself, you are likely to feel the need to question or challenge the practice of others in your workplace. We are often threatened by being challenged, particularly if it is unexpected or at the wrong time or in the wrong place, and in some cases we may be defensive.

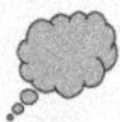

During a normal working day, consider what your reaction would be if a colleague, student or practice assessor/mentor challenged you on why you were doing something in a certain way.

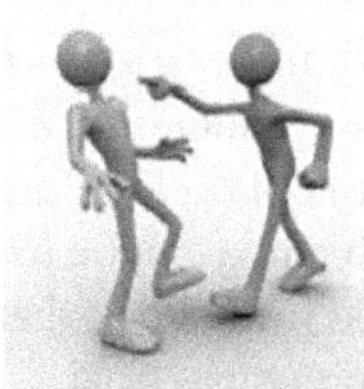

Figure 5.2

How you can reduce the need to challenge the practice of others

Where possible, reduce the need to challenge others by being proactive in your approach:

- Agree a regular time slot such as team meetings, case presentations or handovers when practice decisions and rationale can be discussed.
- Invite students/colleagues to question you (appropriately) and let them know how and when to do this.
- Encourage any new staff and students to share with you any new ideas, information/evidence they may have.
- Either pick a small and easily researched area to focus on first; *or*
- Consider some larger issue that may have inconsistent or unclear rationale and identify what the available evidence is in relation to it.
- Practise 'thinking out loud' to each other to share your rationale and decision-making in a safe and supportive way.

Try to adopt any of the approaches above next time you are working.

Tactfully challenging or questioning the practice of others

Don't forget that it is easier to challenge or question practice if you also regularly *offer praise* when you see good practice. The following are some general tips:

- Ask others for their perspective on the issue/your observations.
- Consider asking questions rather than making accusations.
- Consider whether the practice is unsafe or inappropriate and what your role might be as an advocate for your patients/clients. Addressing the issue becomes urgent if unsafe practice is observed.
- Before you challenge the practice of others, consider whether you have all the evidence you need – are there things you might be unaware of, for example, context, more than one approach or different personal/professional values?
- Access and supply evidence to support your argument or perspective before you challenge others (e.g. showing someone the guidance or policy).
- Consider the setting: avoid challenging another professional in public unless the practice is unsafe. Ask to speak to them privately.
- Assess risk – you should not delay if anyone is putting others at risk. *You should seek guidance on this from your professional body.*
- Give them opportunity and time to respond; people are often more defensive if they are expected to respond immediately. Listen to their perspective.
- Think carefully about the words you use. For example: '*Why are you doing it that way?*' sounds rather like an accusation, whereas '*I haven't seen it done like that before, I'd be interested in knowing if there are any reasons for that approach*' sounds more like an enquiry and is therefore less threatening.

Raising and escalating concerns about practice

There may be instances when, depending on the issue, you may need to raise concerns in a more formal way. You should raise your concern first with the person in question and then with your line manager. Your organization or professional body may stipulate who you should go to next. This process is often called 'escalating concerns'. We have discussed accountability earlier in this book and part of being an accountable professional is identifying and raising concerns if we see or hear about unsafe practice. To avoid 'whistleblowers', teams should adopt a pro-active approach to avoiding unsafe practice.

In the UK, the Nursing and Midwifery Council (NMC 2023b) has produced guidelines for nurses and midwives [https://www.nmc.org.uk/standards/guidance/raising-concerns-guidance-for-nurses-and-midwives/]. Remember that if others see you practising in an unsafe way, then these may apply to you. The Health and Care Professions Council (HCPC 2018) also has guidance for raising and escalating concerns in the workplace and this is available on their website [https://www.hcpc-uk.org.uk/concerns/raising-concerns/].

Using questions to develop a more in-depth approach to critical thinking

Once you have embraced some of the ideas for critical thinking outlined in the earlier part of this chapter, you may want to develop a more *in-depth* approach to thinking critically. You may want to consider Brookfield's (2012) four key questions for critical thinking:

1. What assumptions am I making about the situation or topic?
2. How can I check out these assumptions for accuracy and truth?
3. What alternative perspectives are there?
4. What action should I take following my analysis?

For specific information/evidence that you see, hear or read, you could then apply the '**Six questions for critical thinking**' (see Chapter 1).

Questions to ask when thinking about challenging situations

Delany et al. (2013) conducted a survey of experienced professionals to determine what questions they asked when thinking about a challenging patient/client situation. We have adapted them below for more general situations. Delany et al. placed them into three categories which relate clearly to definitions given earlier of 'evidence-based practice' that include research evidence, judgement and patient/client preferences:

1   **Professional/clinical role**
   - What is the scope of my role?
   - What is the scope of my practice?
   - Is it appropriate for me to be involved?

1
- Should I accept or decline this referral?
- What options do I have to treat these problems?
2 **Knowledge**
- What can I see?
- What does not look right or not normal?
- How does this deviate from normal?
- What information/evidence do I have or what do I know about this condition/situation?
- What information/evidence or knowledge do I need?
- What knowledge do I have access to?
- How would I acquire extra knowledge about this condition/situation?
- Where can I get more information/evidence?
- Who or what can provide this knowledge?
- How can I confirm this knowledge is correct/reliable?
3 **Patient/client perspective: professional reasoning questions based on the patient/client narrative and context**
- What symptoms/problems does the patient/client present with?
- What effect is this having on their activities/life?
- What are the patient's/client's goals?

More 'questions for critical thinking in practice'

In addition to the above, we have developed the following detailed table: **'Questions for critical thinking in practice'** (drawn from a variety of sources including: Paul and Elder 2005; Huckabay 2009; Golding 2011; Facione 2013). It should help you to think critically about the complexities of professional practice. The questions may help you to consider issues that you come across in practice settings. The second section relates to gathering information/evidence and is probably the most important, as in our busy professional lives we may be pressured into making decisions before we have gained sufficient information/evidence.

Questions for critical thinking in practice

1 **Diagnosing and assessing problems or issues/setting goals or objectives**
- What is the problem or question and is it clearly stated?
- Do you understand the complexity of the issue?

- Could you assess the cause of the actual or potential problem?
- Are you picking up relevant cues (e.g. reading body language or more subtle information)?
- Can you invite others to question your practice and share with you if they have seen different approaches to the same issue/problem?
- What are your motivations for changing or challenging this aspect of practice?
- Do you need to ask further questions of your patients/clients/colleagues to get a fuller picture?
- Are you open to the possibility that you may be wrong?
- If setting goals, are they relevant and clearly stated?
- How will you judge the effectiveness of your decisions and interventions?

2   **Gathering information/evidence and further assessment**
- Can you define key ideas/issues?
- Consider the '**Six questions for critical thinking**', **Questions 1** and **2**.
- Have you searched for the best available information/evidence? Could you consider using decision analysis tools to identify your options (e.g. Banning 2008) or ethical reasoning frameworks (e.g. Seedhouse 2009)?
- Do you need to categorize, using frameworks or scales (e.g. risk assessment tools)?
- Can you identify what is objective and what is subjective about your reasoning?
- Do you have enough information/evidence on which to form a reasonable opinion?
- Do you need to ask yourself and others if there is anything else to consider?

3   **Evaluating the evidence**
- Consider the '**Six questions for critical thinking**', **Questions 3, 4, 5** and **6**.
- Make sure you understand all the evidence you have.
- Have you judged the credibility and strength of the arguments presented and are they convincing?
- How significant is the information/evidence?
- Is all the evidence relevant? Reject anything that isn't.
- Can you compare or contrast perspectives?

4   **Reaching conclusions/implementing**
- Consider all '**Six questions for critical thinking**' and the final section: **So what?** (see Figure 2.1).

- What are the implications and consequences of your findings?
- What conclusions might you draw?
- Have you got enough information/evidence?
- Have you considered whether any bias, prejudices or emotions have impacted on your conclusions? For example, might you make a decision to act in a certain way based on what it might involve you having to do?
- Are your conclusions relevant to the context in which you are working?
- Have you considered the implications of these conclusions for others?
- What might you need to consider regarding implementing your findings?

5   **Giving rationale for actions/sharing with colleagues**
- Could you give a clear rationale for your decisions?
- Could you explain to your employers, professional body, colleagues and clients why you acted, or decided not to act, in a situation or set of circumstances?
- Have you documented your reasons?
- Could you explain why you rejected alternative actions or approaches?
- If you are facilitating the learning of others (e.g. colleagues, students or patients/clients), are you presenting the information/evidence in a way that they will easily understand?

Examples of critical thinking in practice

To illustrate how you can incorporate our '**Six questions for critical thinking**' or some of above questions into your daily practice in a more practical way, we will now provide some examples of how you can think more critically about the issues in question.

Example 1: Thinking critically about what you write

Take the statement 'We deliver person-centred care'. A team of professionals may plan to incorporate this into written material they provide to clients about their service. However, without some critical thinking by all concerned, the statement could be interpreted differently by different people or really have little value. To avoid any misinterpretation and make it relevant, the team could:

- Discuss their reasons for wanting to adopt the statement.
- Access any relevant frameworks or guidance on 'person-centred care'.
- Explore what the team's interpretation of 'person-centred care' is. This may involve discussion and searching the literature. They then may want to agree (as a team) an acceptable definition (or indeed write a new one) to use in their publication. It then becomes much more explicit and so can be applied and interpreted better by staff.
- Discuss and explore with patients/clients/stakeholders any potential areas of conflict in applying the concept of 'person-centred care' in advance of adopting it in their written material.
- Clearly discuss and identify what delivering 'person-centred care' will mean in practice and how it will influence ways of working with patients/clients.

Example 2: Thinking critically about what you see

Imagine that you do not know how to handle a particular professional or clinical issue, but you observe a senior and respected colleague dealing with such a situation in a particular way. Before adopting their approach, you could:

- Clarify with your colleague the nature of the issue or problem.
- Discuss with your colleague their reasons for the approach they took.
- Ask them if there is any evidence and evaluate it.
- Discuss with other colleagues if there are any alternative approaches.
- Decide what practice to adopt.

Example 3: Thinking critically about sources of evidence you may hear or read about

A student/colleague rather reluctantly says they have seen you carry out a particular intervention differently from how they have seen it done before. You could:

- Invite the student/colleague to discuss different practices they have seen.
- Ask if they searched for or have access to any additional information/evidence relating to the approach(es) they have seen previously.

- Justify your reasons for your own approach to the intervention and see if and how your reasons are similar or different from theirs.
- With the student/colleague, search for and appraise the 'best available evidence' related to how to perform the skill.
- Proactively continue to discuss with the student/colleague the intervention in order to identify whether there are inconsistencies in the approach and then together you can agree and adopt 'best practice'.

From the questions and examples, you can see that a wide range of skills are needed to be a critical thinker. But many of them can be incorporated into your work, requiring little extra time.

Critical thinking in practice is key to providing safe and effective evidence-based care. It is not satisfactory to work as a professional without questioning yourself and others. 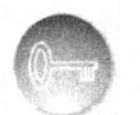

Influencing the 'critical thinking' culture of your workplace

It may be difficult to more broadly influence professional practice if you are the only 'critical thinker' in the workplace! We now offer some 'top tips' for influencing those you work with in order to change the culture of your workplace to a 'learning organization'. The Social Care Institute for Excellence (accessed 2024) has an online resource pack that is designed to allow organizations to assess whether they are learning organizations – that is, organizations that use evidence-based practice and informed decision-making.

'Top tips' for influencing your organizational culture to develop a more critical approach to professional practice

- Find out who the most positive and influential people are (it may not be the people at the top!).
- With these positive influential people on your side, talk to your managers and colleagues, or your mentor, about what makes a learning organization and how you can develop a more critical approach to professional practice.

- Identify those who are reluctant to adopt a questioning and learning approach, and try and find out what their concerns are. You may need to help them see the benefits of safe and effective patient/client care.
- Find out what areas of practice in your workplace are inconsistent or frustrating for your colleagues/learners (see previous sections of this chapter).
- Ask students or visitors to your workplace what practices they have seen performed differently in other areas or with other professionals.
- Involve and encourage your colleagues/students in developing a critical approach to practice.
- The move towards becoming a 'learning organization' will not happen overnight and you may need to make small changes, one at a time.

In summary

In this chapter, we have shown that to be accountable, we need to demonstrate critical thinking in order to be safe and effective. We have looked at the complexities of professional life and explored the pros and cons of basing your practice on routine, experience, using professional judgement and learning from others. We have identified three ways you can start to incorporate critical thinking into your professional practice: using reflection; identifying which aspects of your practice may need to change; and seeking out evidence for professional practice and discussing this within your team. We then considered how to develop more in-depth approaches to critical thinking using questions, before finally exploring how to identify and promote a critical approach in your organization.

Key points

1   Critical thinking is more complex in professional practice than in academic writing or presenting.
2   Many factors affect our practice, including following routine, relying on experience and the influence of others.

3   You can start to think more critically by reflecting on your practice and by considering your practice and the evidence you use to underpin it.
4   Asking questions will help you to facilitate deeper critical thinking within professional practice.
5   It is useful to identify whether your workplace/placement has a critical approach to learning and consider how to influence it.

6 Shaping the future: what is the role of critical thinking in the development of health and social care services?

- *Why is critical thinking important for developing a broader perspective in your personal, professional and academic life?*
- *What are the changes influencing health and social care in the twenty-first century, and how can critical thinking help you to respond to these?*
- *How can you think more critically about these changes?*

> • *Skills and qualities needed to promote critical thinking in relation to broader perspectives in health and social care*
> • *Broadening your horizons in health and social care in your academic work and practice*
> • *In summary*
> • *Key points*

In this chapter, we will:

- Explore why critical thinking is important for developing a broader perspective in your personal, professional and academic life.
- Discuss the changes influencing health and social care in the twenty-first century and explore ways to respond to these as a critical thinker.
- Describe what qualities and skills are needed to think critically from a broader perspective in relation to health and social care.
- Discuss how you can broaden your horizons through networking with professionals and academics in different disciplines, professions and specialist fields.

Why is critical thinking important for developing a broader perspective in your personal, professional and academic life?

As stated in previous chapters, there is no point in being able to demonstrate your skills of critical thinking in the classroom or in your academic work if it ultimately makes no difference to the care you offer to patients and clients.

So far in this book, we have discussed how you can develop your critical thinking skills in relation to your academic work, and in relation to your own practice. A questioning and open-minded approach can contribute not only to the improvement of your academic grades and to the development of your own practice, it can also lead to developments in practice at organizational, regional, national and even international level. It can also influence the development of new theory related to health and social care practice. We now discuss how you can enhance your critical thinking skills by considering broader perspectives that are relevant to health and social care practice.

Influences on your skills of critical thinking

Many factors may have influenced the development – or otherwise – of your skills of critical thinking, including your upbringing, as well as the content and design of any education or training that you have attended, and the teaching/training approaches you have experienced throughout your life. Consideration of these factors may assist you now, as you continue to build on and apply the skills for critical thinking to your academic and professional life.

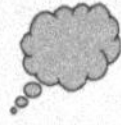

At this point in your life, what do you think have been the key influences – in your day-to-day life, your upbringing and your education – on the development of your skills of critical thinking? Have you been encouraged to question what you read, see and hear? Have you been encouraged to challenge your beliefs, values and assumptions?

Important questions to consider include:

- Did your parents/guardians punish you as a child if you got an answer wrong?
- Throughout your education, were you ever humiliated by a teacher/ lecturer for getting an answer wrong?
- Was asking questions seen as a sign of interest and enthusiasm, or was it discouraged?
- Were you encouraged to be 'seen and not heard'?
- Have you been encouraged by teachers to question, challenge and debate what you were being taught?
- Have you been encouraged to explore and find things out for yourself?
- In your professional training and/or career, have you been encouraged to consider and suggest new ways of working? Have those around you been willing to consider change and/or challenges to their practice?

When considering these questions, you may begin to recognize how your previous experiences – personal, academic and/or professional – may have influenced your approach and attitude to critical thinking.

Many writers have argued that in recent years, in further and higher professional education in many countries, there has been an emphasis on the development of specific skills, focusing on the development of 'competence' and 'employability' (Bridges 2000; Brunt 2005; Gallacher and Osborne 2005). Generally, these terms relate to the mastery of 'instrumental' skills and related knowledge, such as the development of specific practical skills and procedures required for a particular professional role, or of skills related to numeracy or information technology. However, many authors argue that developing 'higher-order' skills such as critical thinking, including the skills required to respond effectively to change, to manage complex situations, to appraise information, and to make judgements and choices, is extremely important in the education of health and social care professionals. In this chapter, we argue that thinking critically should be an endless process in the changing world that health and social care professionals are a part of.

Indeed, some academics even argue that students in higher education should be encouraged to consider broader issues, such as ethics, political issues, sustainability and environmental issues related to their field of study, in order to understand their practice and studies in a wider context. They maintain that taking a wider perspective prepares students to think more broadly, to be more culturally sensitive, and to be better able to deal with complex problems and challenges in a critical manner.

We therefore believe that a focus on specific facts, skills and procedures and on a competency-based approach to professional education leads to a narrowing of students' educational experiences. This is why it can be frustrating to be told as a student (or at any stage of your career!), 'This is how it is done', without any opportunity for discussion or debate.

In professional education there should be an emphasis on developing creative and flexible professionals who are able to think critically, question and respond effectively to rapid change.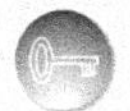

Brookfield (2012), who had a lifetime career exploring the role of critical thinking in professional life, suggests that the ability to think critically is essential in our working life, contending that health and social care professionals should be equipped not merely with information and skills to ensure their competence concerning practice-based skills, but also with the following skills and qualities:

- Skills for critical thinking.
- The ability to reflect on issues and incidents.
- Flexibility, including the ability to consider different viewpoints and approaches.
- The ability to challenge their own assumptions and ways of thinking.

What are the changes influencing health and social care in the twenty-first century, and how can critical thinking help you to respond to these?

Being a critical thinker has never been so important in the fast-changing, flexible and responsive world we live in. Many changes taking place at local, national and global level are impacting significantly on the planning and delivery of health and social care in the twenty-first century. These are leading to new opportunities for positive change, but also to a variety of challenges. It is worth taking stock of these changes, as they will affect your role as a health and social care professional in the future, as well as your future studies and research.

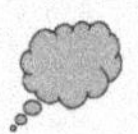

What changes are you are aware of that are taking place locally, nationally and globally that are impacting on the planning and delivery of health and social care in the twenty-first century?

You may have thought of some or all of the following:

- Advances in information access and communication technology.
- Increasing diversity of populations.
- Limitations in financial and material resources to provide health and social care.
- Inequalities in health and in social well-being.
- Political changes, including changes in policy at local, national and international level.
- Environmental issues.
- Globalization.

Advances in information access and communication technology

As discussed in Chapter 1, advances in technology and communication, particularly those related to the development of the internet, have led to increasingly sophisticated ways of accessing information and to the development of many new forms of communication. These have led to dramatic changes in how knowledge and information can be transferred, and how people can interact.

Increasing access to a wide range of information from different disciplines offers health and social care professionals the opportunity to broaden and update their knowledge and apply this new knowledge to their practice. Professional knowledge in health and social care is developing constantly. As we discussed in Chapter 1, keeping up to date with all the information available to us, and knowing how to make the most of it, can seem overwhelming. As practitioners accountable for their own actions, health and social care professionals may find it challenging to keep abreast of rapid changes in theory, research and practice. In addition, patients/clients now have access to information about services, conditions and treatments, making many of them more informed and 'expert' in relation to their care, potentially leading them to have higher expectations of the care and treatment they receive. This can therefore lead to challenges for health and social care professionals.

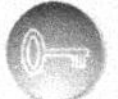

An ever-expanding variety of forms of information technology has also brought new ways to seek, share and store information, offering us new methods for researching issues that may be encountered in our studies and practice.

A wider choice of avenues of communication can be advantageous for many reasons. First, growing networks of communication enable the rapid dissemination of knowledge, including research findings, leading to the potential for more rapid developments in practice and in clinical technology. Secondly, we can communicate in much more flexible ways with others, including professionals and patients/clients, at local and much broader levels, using different forms of communication. For example:

- Emailing other individuals
- Instant messaging
- Online discussion forums

- Chat rooms
- Conferencing software, Microsoft Teams, Zoom, Google Meet
- Wikis
- X (formerly Twitter)
- Email discussion groups.

These can all provide the opportunity for networking among students, practitioners and researchers in order to share knowledge and expertise. Clients can also use these forms of communication as means of finding out about services and obtaining advice and information. However, keeping up to date with rapid developments in communication technology, and knowing how to make the most of these and how to use them can be challenging, and as a health or social care student/professional you need to think critically about their use.

In summary, rapidly advancing technology offers many opportunities for developments in communication, research and practice. You will, however, need to think critically about what forms of communication you choose to use, and which sources of information are available to you to access.

Increasing diversity of populations

Planning and delivering services to suit the needs of a population, whether at a local level or more broadly, can prove challenging. As a result of globalization, population migration and a variety of social factors, most populations throughout the world have become increasingly diverse in relation to, for example, culture, age and ethnicity. For example, the 2021 census in England and Wales indicated a rise in ethnic and racial diversity, with increased numbers of mixed-heritage children, increased numbers of older people from minority backgrounds, and concentrations of people from different ethnic and racial backgrounds in particular cities, such as Birmingham and London (ONS 2022). The population of England and Wales was also shown to have a significantly higher proportion of older people than in 2001, and other changes were highlighted, including a significant increase in the proportion of people who stated that they have no religious affiliation. Such changes pose new challenges in terms of how health and welfare services are planned to meet the needs of different localities.

From a wider perspective, according to the United Nations (2009), significant population ageing is occurring in most countries worldwide;

this again has a major impact on demands for health and social care services as well as on economic growth, consumption and labour markets, and will influence family composition and epidemiology. In the political arena, this may in turn influence voting patterns and political representation. Increasing population diversity will therefore have many potential implications for planning health and social care services in different populations – locally, nationally and globally.

Health and social care professionals have had to respond to – and think critically about – the increasing diversity of populations, ensuring that appropriate services are planned and delivered appropriately, taking the diversity of clients within a local population into account. They therefore need to understand different worldviews and appreciate the complexity of notions of culture and the increasing interconnectedness between different nations and cultures throughout the world (Department of Health 2009; Harrison and Melville 2010; Holland 2010). The professional regulatory bodies governing and guiding health and social care practice in the UK, such as the Nursing and Midwifery Council and the Health and Care Professions Council, highlight that it is vital to understand and respect different perspectives, values and worldviews, appreciating the complexities of different cultures and recognizing how intercultural issues may be relevant to professional practice – this is likely to become even more important as populations become increasingly diverse. Oozageer Gunowa et al. (2021) explored the way in which pressure injury care was taught to pre-registration nursing students with a specific focus on whether the effects of skin damage on people with different skin tones was part of the teaching delivered. Despite much discussion about the need for inclusive teaching, Oozageer Gunowa et al. did not find an inclusive approach and identified that nurse education, at the time of the study, was taught based on the assumption that the recipients of care would have white skin. Health and social care professionals are responsible for educating the next generation of health and social care practitioners, where it is critical to model diversity in professional practice.

The number of autistic university students is increasing (Gillespie-Lynch et al. 2020), including among pre-registration health and social care students. This may be a situation that readers of this book may identify with and the issue of seeking perfection in your critical writing. It is important to work with your tutors and university support services so that you can identify your strengths and successfully develop your critical thinking and writing.

Limitations in financial and material resources to provide health and social care

Although patterns of public spending vary widely across different countries, health and social care practitioners working in all settings are likely to have finite resources – both financial and material – available to them when planning and delivering services. As a result, they may need to make difficult choices regarding how best to meet the needs of the populations they serve (Blakemore and Griggs 2007; Alcock and May 2014). Spending has to be reviewed on a regular basis; changing budgets and blurring between health and social care services may lead to difficult decisions regarding the funding of services, such as home care and day centres, reduced funding for which will remove support for older people. Cuts of this type may lead to the development of more health and social problems in the long term.

Health and social care professionals may have to justify their requests for more funding for resources or services; at other times, they may be able to make creative suggestions for more effective ways to use limited resources, financial or otherwise, based on their experiences in practice or on research findings. At times health and social care professionals might need to speak up for resources they need to ensure their own safety. For example, Ayres (2023) explored how when assaults are committed against mental health nurses, these are often not addressed, given the resources that would be required to do so. Instead, nurses are encouraged to put on a 'brave face' and return to the workplace as if nothing untoward had occurred. Ayres recommends that resources are put in place for safeguarding the needs of mental health nurses. Critical thinking skills are therefore essential to ensure that effective care is provided in a way that is responsive to both clients' and professionals' needs, taking into account any constraints in relation to funding and resources.

Inequalities in health and in social well-being

Some differences in health status between individuals are biological in origin, linking to age and genetic differences. However, many disparities in population health and social well-being between social groups, and also between nations, are largely societal in origin. They are influenced by the way societies are organized along social, economic and political lines and reflect the powerful stratifying forces that differentiate life opportunities and social need, both within and between countries. The United Nations/WHO (UNEP/WHO 2008) have long observed that there are dramatic inequalities in health within and between countries that are closely linked with degrees of social disadvantage. Similarly, in 2022 the Office for National Statistics census data acknowledged that health inequalities in the UK between rich and poor were widening, and that certain conditions that were increasing, such as childhood obesity, are linked closely to social inequalities. Aiming to promote social justice and reduce health inequalities globally, the United Nations Foundation introduced the Sustainable Development Goals (SDGs) in 2015. These 17 goals aim to provide a blueprint to deliver a sustainable and more equitable world for everyone and focus on climate change, reducing poverty, and improving education, health and economic growth. The goals that are most pertinent within health and social care include promoting health and well-being (SDG 3) and reduced inequality (SDG 10), although arguably all the SDGs have a relevance to the wider interests in health and social care (United Nations, undated).

Health and social care professionals, and all those who plan health and social care services, may have to respond to inequalities in health and social well-being at local, national and global level, and may be involved in making difficult decisions about how care is to be rationed. Critical thinking is essential in order to respond to such challenges effectively. An example of this would be the difficult decisions that had to be taken during the COVID-19 epidemic regarding the allocation of resources and the assessment not only of those most in need but also of those who would obtain maximum benefit.

Political changes, including changes in policy at local, national and international level

Political changes at local, national and global level will impact on how health and social care services are planned, funded and run. It is therefore important that those working in the fields of health and social care have a critical awareness of how policies are created and reviewed, and that they are able to critically appraise existing policy and analyse proposals for new policy.

Health and social care professionals may be involved in the process of formulating policy, either formally or informally. An understanding of current affairs in health and social policy, and an involvement in shaping policy, can therefore be an important aspect of a professional's role.

Clients/service users/patients and carers are having an increasing role in shaping developments in many health and social care services, to ensure that their perspectives are taken into account.

An example from the UK of when current affairs have influenced health and social care policy and practice is the impact of the investigation into issues relating to management and delivery of care within the Mid Staffordshire NHS Foundation Trust, which is still affecting policy one decade later. A report summarizing the issues raised during this investigation (Francis 2013) has led to a wide range of recommendations for new management practices and for changes in how NHS care is organized and delivered, in order to promote higher quality care for patients, prioritizing their safety and well-being. This report has had a considerable impact on the work of those working in NHS services at all levels.

It is essential that people working in health and social care services remain alert to issues relating to their own practice and keep abreast of current affairs and of recommendations for changes in policy and practice in order to remain accountable for their practice. Health and social care professionals should read policies and recommendations for practice with a critical eye. They should also observe whether proposals set out in policies, at local, regional, national or international level, are always translated into practice.

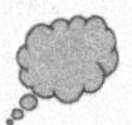

What might be potential barriers to the recommendations set out in policies (e.g. national or local) becoming translated into practice in health and social care services? How should health and social care professionals act if they are responsible for implementing recommendations but are faced with such barriers?

Environmental issues

There is increasing acknowledgement of the impact of environmental issues, at both local and wider levels, on individuals' and populations' health and social well-being. As long ago as 1987 the United Nations stated that, 'All human beings have the fundamental right to an environment adequate for their health and well-being.' More recently, the Royal College of Nursing published a statement on responding to climate change (RCN 2019), emphasizing that initiatives that are good for the wider environment are also good for the health of the individual.

The impacts of climate change have long been understood. As long ago as 2011, the World Health Organization (WHO 2011) was highlighting the impact of environmental factors on death and disease, stating that environmental hazards are responsible for around a quarter of the total burden of disease worldwide, and that in the developing world one-third of death and disease is the result of environmental factors. The WHO also suggested that in developed countries, healthier environments could significantly reduce the incidence of cancers, cardiovascular disease, asthma, lower respiratory infections, musculoskeletal diseases, road traffic injuries, poisonings and drowning. Policy-makers at local, national and global level may be charged with tackling issues related to environmental sustainability and climate change, and with monitoring how these factors may impact on the health and social well-being of populations.

Since then, there have been global initiatives to minimize the effects of climate change and its corresponding effects on health care. For example, Romanello et al. (2023) report on the expertise of scientists and health professionals who have assessed the potential impact of climate change. Reducing the impact of climate change is dependent on achieving commitment from those who will be affected by any action. In a large international survey, Kotcher et al. (2021) explore the views of health professionals on climate change. The authors report that despite a high level of awareness of the need for action, the majority of participants described a range of barriers preventing them taking action themselves and call for a joint response for action on climate change to prevail.

Globalization

The growing speed and intensity of global interactions due to the broadening of social, political and economic activities across political frontiers, regions and continents mean that the effects of distant events can be highly significant elsewhere and potentially have enormous global consequences (Held et al. 1999). As a result, there is an ever-increasing interdependence between different communities around the world – what happens to one community will have implications for others, at all levels, locally, nationally and globally (Harrison and Melville 2010). For example, economic issues in one country will impact on others around the world; and environmental issues in one region will affect those around it, whether locally or more widely. Those planning and delivering health and social care services therefore need to understand the wider context of their work, making connections between local and global events and issues.

How can you think more critically about these changes?

There is clearly a need for health and social care professionals to respond to the above changes, taking into account broader perspectives when planning and delivering care and services.

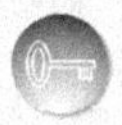

*A broader view is needed, beyond a focus on the care of individuals and on one's own profession and specialism. This requires a **critical perspective**.*

Below is a framework that can help you identify which broader issues may influence health and social care for individuals and communities. Dahlgren and Whitehead (1993) were commissioned by the World Health Organization to identify the social determinants of health upon which public health policy could be based.

Dahlgren and Whitehead's (1993) model remains widely used today. The model outlined a thought-provoking 'rainbow model' depicting the 'social determinants of health' (see Figure 6.1), suggesting that there is a

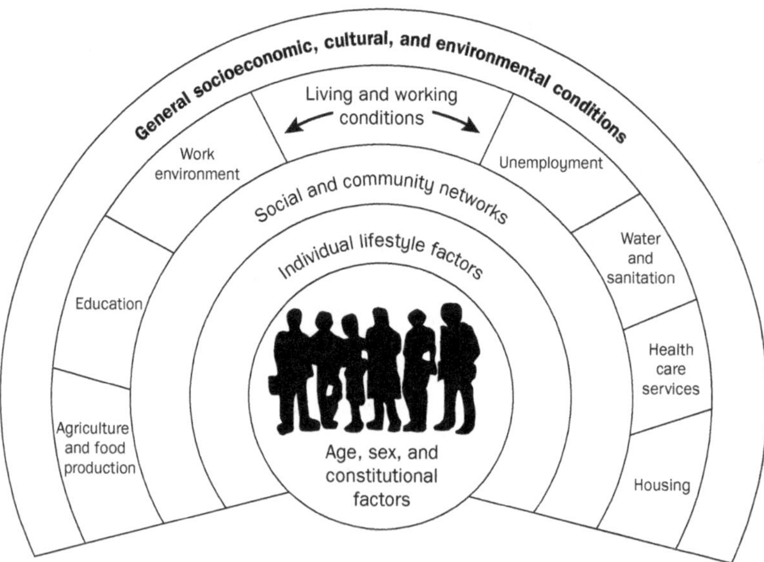

Figure 6.1 The social determinants of health (Dahlgren and Whitehead 1993, 2007)

strong relationship between the individual, their environment, social factors and their health status. They saw the individual (e.g. client/patient or family) as being *at the centre*, with a set of fixed factors (e.g. genetic make-up, age and sex) impacting on their health that cannot be changed. Perhaps in our professional practice these are the first things we notice when we assess our patients/clients. Surrounding them, however, are 'layers of influence' that affect the health of individuals in populations – these can be modified, and it is perhaps these broader issues that we should think more critically about as we assess and plan the care for our patients/clients and their families.

First, an individual's personal behaviour and their ways of living can either promote or damage their health. For example, an individual may choose to smoke tobacco or drink alcohol, both of which are likely to impact negatively on their health. Dahlgren and Whitehead suggest that targeted health promotion aiming to influence individuals' lifestyles and attitudes may be an effective strategy to improve the health and well-being of individuals and communities.

Secondly, Dahlgren and Whitehead (1993) suggest that a person's well-being will also be affected by their social support network, such as their family, friends and community networks. They suggest that strengthening community support could be an effective way to improve the health and well-being of individuals and populations.

Thirdly, Dahlgren and Whitehead suggest that structural factors, such as housing, access to employment, working conditions, access to services and to essential facilities (e.g. sanitation and clean water), will also influence an individual's health and how they respond to ill health. They thus argue that improving living and working conditions will have a positive impact on the health and well-being of individuals and communities.

Finally, the authors suggest that broader factors – socioeconomic, cultural and environmental – can also impact on an individual's health. They suggest that attention should be given to these factors and to how ill-health can be prevented through focusing on them as well as the 'inner layers' of the 'rainbow'. This reflects some of the broader issues we have been exploring in this chapter.

As this model clearly illustrates, we need to think more critically about all these issues when assessing and planning health and social care for individuals and communities. You could use this model alongside either the '**Six questions for critical thinking**' from Chapter 1 or the '**Questions for critical thinking in practice**' from Chapter 5, as prompts to help you to think more broadly about issues you wish to analyse in your studies or in relation to your practice.

Skills and qualities needed to promote critical thinking in relation to broader perspectives in health and social care

As a result of the changes and challenges outlined above, professionals will be expected to have skills and qualities to enable them to work flexibly, as reflective and adaptable team players, able to deal with the increasingly complex issues that may be encountered in health and social care practice. This requires skills of critical thinking.

In the earlier chapters of this book, we have discussed some of the approaches that characterize critical thinking, including *inquisitiveness* in relation to a wide range of issues, *flexibility* when considering alternatives and opinions, and *open-mindedness* regarding divergent world-views.

To improve your understanding of diversity of populations, you could seek out and take up any opportunity to learn with, from and about other professionals and service users in a variety of communities, cultures and countries. If you have the opportunity to take part in an exchange system to go abroad, or to experience working in new environments, you should consider participating in such activities.

In addition to the qualities and skills required for critical thinking discussed in previous chapters, there are other qualities and skills needed to incorporate broader issues that will help you to work positively in a rapidly changing and unpredictable health and social care environment. These are as follows:

- *Flexibility*: as health and social care professionals, you need to be reflective and adaptable team players, able to deal with the complex issues you will encounter in your practice. You need to be flexible in your thinking, open-minded, able to question your own values and assumptions, and able to question what you read, see and hear.
- *Creativity*: this will assist the development of new approaches to your practice, studies and research. A creative approach is needed to your own practice in order to tackle the issues you face.
- *Sound coping strategies*: these are required to assist you to cope positively with complexity, uncertainty and unpredictability (Barnett 2000, 2004).
- *Responsiveness*: this will enable you to respond appropriately to rapid changes and developments in health and social care practice.

Expanding on these, the following skills and qualities will be invaluable if you wish to develop your skills of critical thinking within your practice and within your studies:

- **A willingness to question the breadth of your own knowledge about health and social care:** it is important to recognize that you may have a narrow viewpoint, if you have no knowledge or experience of other cultures. For example, you may have beliefs about bereavement that are related to your own culture, or you may select research that was carried out in a culture similar to your own rather than looking for broader perspectives on the topic.
- **A willingness to engage with students and professionals from overseas who may be working with you:** there are likely to be many differences between your own and their practices. Promote positive debate about why these differences exist, and encourage an atmosphere where people can learn 'with, from and about' each other, sharing good practice.
- **A willingness to reflect upon and think critically about how your beliefs and values influence your professional decision-making:** acknowledge that your beliefs will be influenced by many factors, including your culture, gender, age, and social and economic circumstances – be prepared to question and challenge them.
- **An openness to new ideas and perspectives from a diverse range of people:** be willing to actively listen to different viewpoints and theories and to consider their merits, even when they are different from your own. For example, when researching a topic, you could consider pieces of research undertaken in a variety of cultures, to compare these with what you find in your own culture.
- **The ability and willingness to work effectively** in environments that are international and intercultural in nature – developing skills to work effectively with people from different cultures and nationalities and care sensitively for people from different cultures and nationalities.
- **The ability to interpret local problems within a broad, international and intercultural context**, taking into account different perspectives in relation to issues and problems.
- **A broader questioning approach, including:**
  - Questioning what you read, see or hear, taking into account the cultural influences, the setting and/or other potential background influences.

- The ability and willingness to recognize and to question your own and others' potential agendas and biases.

Broadening your horizons in health and social care in your academic work and practice

Thinking critically about health and social care issues from a wider viewpoint can help you to gain new perspectives and develop your own and others' practice. It could also lead to higher grades in your academic work.

Linking to broader perspectives in your academic work

Depending on the focus of your studies, ways to link to broader perspectives in your academic work may include:

- Consideration of the issues raised earlier in this chapter within your academic work:
  - Advances in information access and communication technology.
  - Increasing diversity of populations.
  - Limitations in financial and material resources to provide health and social care.
  - Inequalities in health and social well-being.
  - Political changes.
  - Environmental issues.
  - Globalization.
- Researching for information from different disciplines and specialist areas that are relevant to your field of practice or your area of academic focus, in order to identify different factors that can impact on health and social care issues – see Dahlgren and Whitehead's (1993) framework above.
- Researching for information/research from different cultures and backgrounds, including from different countries that you might not normally access, to take into account wider perspectives on your topic.
- Networking with people such as practitioners, specialists, professionals and academics working in your own and other fields, specialities and disciplines, or who are working in different settings, whose expertise may contribute to your area of interest (see later in the chapter for more information on this).
- Accessing as appropriate a wide range of literature and research relevant to your topic, to take account of broader perspectives.

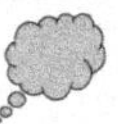

Bearing in mind the above suggestions, consider what approach you might use to research the following question:

What strategies can be used to prevent depression in older people within the UK?

Your initial thoughts may have included the following:

- Access statistics on the prevalence of depression in older people within the UK – for example, see the Office for National Statistics website; search for information in journals/textbooks.
- Carry out a systematic search for textbooks/journal articles on the causes of depression in older people, using the strategies outlined in Chapter 3.
- Undertake a systematic search for textbooks/journal articles on strategies for the prevention of depression in older people in the UK, including relevant policy and guidelines, using the strategies outlined in Chapter 3.
- Carry out a search for relevant websites that may provide high-quality information on the topic, such as those belonging to Age UK, MIND, the Social Care Institute for Excellence (SCIE) and the Department of Health.

Did you think of any other strategies for searching for information, or any other potential sources of information on this topic? If so, what were they?

*Now think more critically about strategies you could use to broaden your search to gain a better perspective on the topic of **the prevention of depression in older people within the UK**. You could use Dahlgren and Whitehead's (1993) framework to help you think about this.*

There are many sources of information that you could refer to in relation to the subject of the prevention of depression in older people in the UK. Alongside the ideas listed above, you could take a broader approach to your search – you may have thought of some ideas already. Some questions that might be useful to ask in order to gain a broader perspective are:

- How does the prevalence of depression in older people in the UK compare with that in other countries globally?
- How does the prevalence of depression in older people vary between different cultural and social groups within the UK? Why might this variation exist?
- Do any cultures have a significantly higher or lower rate of depression in older people than others and, if so, why might that be?
- Are there any strategies that are used successfully in other cultures and countries for preventing depression and promoting well-being in older people? Could these be applied successfully, or adapted, within the UK?
- Why might the prevalence of depression vary between different countries or cultural groups, and what factors may contribute to these variations?
- What policies and guidelines does the current UK government promote? Has this changed, or is it likely to with a change in government?
- Do any other countries have active programmes for preventing depression in older people? If so, what do they consist of, and how effective are they? Could they be applied successfully, or adapted, within the UK?
- What factors beyond your own specialist area of knowledge might be important to consider – medical factors, social factors, economic factors, environmental factors, political factors? How could you search for information on these?

You will, of course, need to *critically appraise and analyse* all the statistics and sources that you read – for example, statistics on depression might not be collected and monitored in the same way in different countries, so it's important to analyse them very carefully. Nevertheless, you may find enlightening information that could help you to view the topic in a different way. This broader approach could help you to widen your perspectives, leading to new ideas that you could apply to your own and others' practice, your academic work and future research.

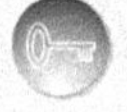

Taking a broader perspective will involve thinking about searching for information from a broader range of sources. However, you need to ensure that you remain focused on your topic or question, as highlighted in Chapter 4.

Having read the above section, consider the wider range of strategies you could use to research one of the following questions:

What are the causes of childhood obesity?

What might be effective strategies for promoting smoking cessation in young adults?

You should have discovered that you can really expand the breadth of information you use in order to gain a broader perspective on the topics you address. We will now offer another way you can widen your horizons – by networking.

Networking

As well as asking broader questions about your topic, you can also widen your knowledge and perspectives relating to a topic by making links with health care practitioners, researchers and service users based in different disciplines, professions, specialities, cultures and countries. These people may be able and willing to share their ideas and perspectives with you in order to shed more light on the issue you are investigating.

You will find many opportunities to communicate with people in order to share ideas and perspectives on topics related to health and social care, on a formal and informal basis, as discussed earlier in the chapter. Thanks to the internet, it is now easier than ever to contact people anywhere in the world to seek their expert knowledge and perspectives. Even if you are unable to meet face-to-face with people easily, such as attending conferences and meetings, you can still use other means such as Skype, email groups, wikis, or joining an online discussion forum.

Within your own discipline, specialty or area of interest, you may have opportunities to join specific networks. For example:

- For the RCN 'Forums and networks' list, see https://www.rcn.org.uk/Get-Involved/Forums-and-networks.
- For details of an international social work network, see www.socialworknetwork.com.

Many professional bodies have interest groups that you can join, and these can provide the starting point for discussions and useful exchange of information and ideas. You may also wish to make more permanent links with other academics and professionals, for example, establishing exchange schemes with people working in different health care systems and different disciplines, so that you can learn with, from and about each other's areas of expertise, sharing good practice.

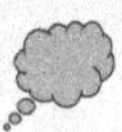

Which disciplines and subject areas could help you to broaden your perspectives in relation to your areas of interest/expertise in health and social care?

You may have thought of some or all of the following: philosophy, ethics, psychology, sociology, life sciences, economics, politics, geography, environmental sciences, forensic medicine, child protection. You may be able to think of others. Sometimes, therefore, you may need to widen your search strategy to look for relevant information from these disciplines and subject areas. You could also consider approaching experts in these fields.

The benefits of networking: a case study

John is an experienced nurse specializing in dermatology (skin care). He has a particular interest in the prevention of skin cancers related to sun exposure. He has had the opportunity to develop his knowledge and skills in a variety of ways:

- He has joined a dermatology interest group in his local area, linking with other professionals with an interest in this topic. They hold regular meetings where they share their knowledge and experiences and have an internet discussion forum through which they can communicate ideas and information.
- He is a member of a national dermatology forum open to practitioners, academics and researchers interested in this topic. They hold regular meetings and an annual national conference where they can share their knowledge, ideas and experiences.
- He is able to contact professionals and academics working in the field of dermatology throughout the world on a day-to-day basis through a variety of means, including emails, online discussion forums and by phone.

- He is also a member of an international dermatology research forum, whose website is updated regularly with the latest developments in research in his specialist field. Every other year, John goes to an international conference organized by this forum, where he can network with professionals from all over the world.
- John can access information via a variety of journals, both national and international, to update his knowledge.
- He has a link with a research centre based in a hospital in Australia that specializes in the prevention and treatment of skin cancers. John has visited the centre three times over the past 10 years, to learn from their good practice and to share his knowledge and experience.
- He also has a link with a hospital in Africa where he has set up an exchange system between their team and his own – they share ideas for how to prevent and treat skin cancers, and benefit from each other's knowledge, experience and ideas.
- John has a developing interest in the impact of genetic factors on the incidence of skin cancer globally, and he is involved in research on this topic with colleagues in the UK, Africa and Australia. The team members have fed back their initial findings to the various forums and interest groups they are involved with locally, nationally and globally. They have written a variety of papers on the prevention of skin cancer aimed at a global audience, which has led to positive changes in the prevention of skin cancer at many levels, and new approaches to researching the issues related to this topic.

John's example illustrates how an individual health or social care practitioner can incorporate broader, global perspectives within their practice, potentially linking these to their studies and research. This can potentially lead to changes in practice and theory at a variety of levels, and requires a creative and questioning approach to practice and research, and openness to alternative ideas and perspectives.

The impact of critical thinking on the development of practice

To sum up the ideas within this chapter, we will conclude with a very short and simple case study that illustrates the potential benefits of critical thinking, combined with broader perspectives in relation to health and social care.

Case study

A motivated inter-professional team of health and social care professionals was involved in running a large nursing home for the long-term care of older people with dementia. Some staff felt increasingly concerned by the number of clients who appeared to be bored and restless during the daytime. Client and carer surveys suggested a low level of satisfaction with care in relation to the mental stimulation of clients in the home.

The team decided to explore how they could improve the care offered. Their lead manager was fully supportive of their plans, and encouraged them to take some time to work on this project, as well as offering a limited amount of financial support.

The approach the team decided to take was as follows:

- First, they met together, along with client and carer representatives, and with an expert in dementia care who was based at their local university. They shared their initial concerns, and discussed their ideas for how they could enhance the care on offer. Each person present discussed how he or she felt they could contribute to the project.
- Two members of the team offered to carry out a thorough search for research, articles and reports highlighting recommendations for good practice. Through this they identified a variety of sources of information, which they critically appraised in order to decide which sources were relevant to their setting. They put together a summary of the key findings of their review to present to the team.
- Other members of the team joined an international online discussion forum for professionals caring for people with dementia. They posted a request for suggestions for improving their practice. A lively debate ensued, and as a result they engaged in live discussions with professionals working in a variety of countries, including the USA, Bolivia, India and Sweden. They received some constructive suggestions from all of these people, who suggested many ideas for how they could enhance client care, including:
  - Involving clients in day-to-day activities around the home.
  - Staff, clients and carers sharing mealtimes, to promote more social interaction.
  - Using new approaches for assessing clients' interests and past histories in more depth.

- o   Using simple ways to engage clients such as the use of music, talking books, etc.; the staff were given useful information about how to access good resources.
- o   Using a variety of simple strategies to communicate with clients more effectively.
- o   Ways of encouraging the local community to become more engaged with people living in the home.
- o   How to decorate and lay out the home in order to enhance clients' sense of freedom, while maximizing their safety.

A year after the first meeting, having introduced these ideas and others, care in the home had improved so significantly that it had become a model for good practice in the local area. Staff from other homes in the region visited to learn from their expertise. One member of the team suggested that they should write an account of the changes they had made, linking to relevant literature, and making recommendations for other professionals contemplating similar changes. The publication of this article in a social care journal led to further developments: staff members working in the home were invited to assist in a Department of Health working party aiming to formulate new standards for dementia care throughout the UK.

One of the people they had been in contact with, who was based in Sweden, asked to visit their home, and an exchange was then arranged. As a result, one of the team had the opportunity to visit some care homes in Sweden. She was able to compare their approaches and share ideas for good practice. While in Sweden, she also gave a presentation at a conference for health and social care professionals, to disseminate good practice, and at the conference she had the opportunity to attend other presentations and learn from dementia care specialists based in different parts of Europe.

In the years following this, the team continued to develop their practice. They were keen to continue to improve their care, and did not 'rest on their laurels'. One member of the team left to set up a consultancy business, with the aim of helping similar homes to enhance their care. As new members of staff joined the home, they fed in their ideas for how to improve and develop care further. The manager continued to foster an open atmosphere whereby staff members were encouraged to develop their knowledge and to share their ideas for good practice, and also to challenge each other's practice in a positive and constructive manner.

This case study highlights the value of working with others who are prepared to challenge their own and others' practice, and illustrates the potential positive effects of thinking critically and seeking ideas from a broader perspective when analysing one's practice. It also shows that academic research feeds into the process of changing practice. It can be extremely fruitful to look further afield beyond one's usual sources of support and information to gain new perspectives on an issue or problem.

'Top tips' for broadening your perspectives in relation to your practice and your academic work

- **Look beyond the reading list:** don't restrict your reading to what is in your reading list! Read more broadly in relation to your topic and, where appropriate, look for information and research from other disciplines, other specialities, other countries and other professions.
- **Ask broader questions of what you read, see and hear:** use the **'Six questions for critical thinking'** from Chapter 1 and the **'Questions for critical thinking in practice'** from Chapter 5 as a basis to help you consider the following questions:
  - Are there any alternative perspectives/viewpoints in relation to the topic/issue you are focusing on?
  - What have different authors/researchers/practitioners/ theorists said – within your own profession/setting/ speciality and in other professions/settings/specialities?
  - What are your own thoughts and ideas, having read different perspectives in research and literature?
  - Do any ethical issues need to be considered? Would the same ethical issues apply elsewhere (e.g. in other countries or settings)?
  - What can you learn from approaches used in other countries and cultures?
  - What can you learn from research carried out in other countries and cultures?
- **Where appropriate, look at broader perspectives related to health and social care:** social, economic, political and/or cultural.
- **Look at other work from other disciplines/specialities** to see what they have to say about the issues you are researching.
- **Become more self-aware:** try to become more aware of your own values, attitudes, beliefs and biases, and think about how these may impact on your thinking and your practice.

- **Make links with other practice areas/specialities:** locally, regionally, nationally, globally – share ideas, learn 'with, from and about' others' approaches to practice issues, including models of health and social care.
- **Discuss issues with peers and colleagues, at the local level and more widely:** this will help you to challenge the taken-for-granted assumptions, beliefs and values that you hold, and to share ideas for developing theory and practice.
- **Consider whether there may be alternative ways of viewing/ approaching the issue or problem you are looking at:** consider your own thoughts, your colleagues' and peers' perspectives, and those of authors and researchers.
- Continually question your knowledge, values and assumptions.

The importance of people exchanging ideas and valuing alternative perspectives to their own cannot be underestimated, and we believe that this is the key to development of practice and the promotion of positive changes in health and social care. Professionals should be equipped to be flexible, creative and innovative thinkers in order to solve problems through questioning. Critical thinkers are more likely to engage in productive and positive activity due to their continual questioning of their knowledge, assumptions and perspectives.

Brookfield (2012) suggests that critical thinking takes place when we do four things:

- **Hunt assumptions** – we need to try to uncover the assumptions that influence the way we think and act. Often, these assumptions are not as accurate as we think they may be, and we need to try to identify what they are.
- **Check assumptions** – once we are aware of the assumptions that influence our actions and thinking, we need to assess whether they are valid and reliable guides for action. We therefore need to look for evidence, through our experiences, through others' guidance, or through credible research/information.
- **See things from different viewpoints** – we need to try to see our assumptions/actions from different points of view: what might other people think about this question/issue? Sometimes it's important to try and see ourselves as others might view us.
- **Take informed action** – having done the three things above, we need to review our actions and take new approaches that are based on

convincing evidence, so that we can explain and justify our actions/ choices/decisions to others.

Critical thinking enables professionals to challenge their own and others' beliefs and habits, and not take things for granted. A critical thinker will look to broader perspectives to help them develop their knowledge, practice and perspectives. This curiosity and open-mindedness will lead to a more rewarding and innovative approach both to your professional practice and to your academic studies.

It is important, however, to remember that critical thinking skills need to be developed over time, and do not always come easily. We hope that this book will help you as you set out on your journey as a critical thinker, in order to enhance your own and others' practice in health and social care in the future.

In summary

In this chapter, we have explored why critical thinking is important for developing a broader perspective in your personal, professional and academic life, noting that there is a need globally for creative and flexible professionals who are able to think critically and respond effectively to rapid change. We have discussed the many changes influencing health and social care in the twenty-first century, and explored how health and social care professionals can respond to these as critical thinkers. We have described the qualities and skills that are needed to think critically from a broader perspective in relation to health and social care. We have also discussed how you can broaden your horizons through networking with professionals and academics in different disciplines, professions and specialist fields.

Key points

1   Thinking critically and taking a broad perspective when analysing theory or practice in relation to health and social care issues can lead to positive developments to your own and others' practice, at local, national and much broader levels, as well as to the development of your academic skills.

2   Health and social care professionals need to be critical thinkers
    to be able to respond effectively to the rapid changes occurring
    in the twenty-first century. A broad perspective is required, taking
    into account the various factors impacting on health and social
    care at local, regional, national and global levels.
3   There are key qualities and skills that will enable you to take a
    broader perspective in relation to your practice and your studies –
    in particular, flexibility, creativity and responsiveness to change.

Appendix: Useful websites

All websites were accessible at the time of writing.

Agency for Healthcare Research & Quality (AHRQ). A public resource for evidence-based clinical practice guidelines [https://www.ahrq.gov/]

Agree Collaboration. An international collaboration of researchers and policy-makers who seek to improve the quality and effectiveness of clinical practice guidelines, by establishing a shared framework for their development, reporting and assessment [http://www.agreetrust.org/]

Bad Science. Author Ben Goldacre discusses many of the myths about health and social care, especially those reported in the media [http://www.badscience.net/]

BMJ Best Practice. An evidence-based patient website, based on the *British Medical Journal*'s Clinical Evidence. It explains chronic conditions and rates the effectiveness of treatments. A subscription is required for access to some information [https://www.bmj.com/company/bmj-resources/bmj-best-practice/]

British Broadcasting Corporation. BBC health news [http://www.bbc.co.uk/news/health/]

Campbell Collaboration. The Campbell Collaboration is an international research network that produces systematic reviews of the effects of social interventions [https://www.campbellcollaboration.org/]

Care Opinion. Care Opinion is about honest and meaningful conversations between patients and health services. They believe that patients' stories can help make health services better [https://www.careopinion.org.uk/]

Centre for Evidence-Based Medicine (CEBM). The aim is to provide all the tools, resources and learning opportunities associated with evidence-based health care [www.cebm.net/]

Centre for Reviews and Dissemination. Provides research-based information about the effects of health and social care interventions via its databases, and undertakes systematic reviews evaluating the research evidence on health and public health questions of national and international importance [http://www.york.ac.uk/inst/crd/]

Citizens Advice. Useful for a wide range of issues/advice [http://www.citizensadvice.org.uk]

Clinical Evidence. An international database of high-quality, rigorously developed systematic overviews assessing the benefits and harms of treatments, and a suite of evidence-based medicine resources and training materials [http://clinicalevidence.bmj.com/ceweb/index.jsp]

Cochrane Collaboration. For systematic reviews, clinical trials and other sources [https://www.cochrane.org]

Cochrane Collaboration Glossary. Provides explanations and definitions of research terms [https://epoc.cochrane.org/sites/epoc.cochrane.org/files/uploads/SURE-Guides-v2.1/Collectedfiles/source/glossary.pdf]

Critical Appraisal Skills Programme (CASP) International. The CASP International Network (CASPin) is an international collaboration that supports the teaching and learning of critical appraisal skills, and in particular helps people set up sustainable training programmes [https://casp-uk.net/]

Critical Thinking Community. The Center for Critical Thinking works under the auspices of the Foundation for Critical Thinking, an educational non-profit organization, to promote essential change in education and society through the cultivation of fair-minded critical thinking. There are a variety of resources and web links but do check the date of some of them [https://www.criticalthinking.org/]

Critical Thinking on the Web. A directory of quality online resources [https://www.reasoninglab.com/ctotw/index.htm]

DISCERN. Ascertains the quality of written information on treatment choices [www.discern.org.uk]

Evidence-Based Answers to Clinical Questions for Busy Clinicians. A workbook published in 2011 (updated 2018) by The Centre for Clinical Effectiveness, Monash Health, Melbourne, Victoria, Australia [https://monashhealth.org/wp-content/uploads/2018/11/Finding-the-Evidence_BusyClinicians2018.pdf]

Foundation for Critical Thinking. A range of video clips on YouTube from key authors in critical thinking [https://www.youtube.com/user/CriticalThinkingOrg]

Health and Care Professions Council (HCPC) [http://www.hcpc-uk.org]

Health and Social Care Information Centre (HSCIC). The trusted national provider of high-quality information, data and IT systems for health and social care [https://digital.nhs.uk/]

Health Information Research Unit (HIRU). Conducts research in the field of health information science and is dedicated to the generation of new knowledge about the nature of health and clinical information problems. Based at the Clinical Epidemiology and Biostatistics Department at McMaster University, Canada, the unit conducts research in the field of health information science [http://hiru.mcmaster.ca/hiru]

Joanna Briggs Institute. Designed to provide you with the best available evidence to inform your clinical decision-making at the point of care [https://jbi.global/]

Mind Tools. A range of information including SWOT analysis [http://www.mindtools.com/pages/article/newTMC_05.htm]

National Institute for Health and Care Excellence (NICE). An independent organization responsible for providing national guidance on promoting good health and preventing and treating ill health [https://www.nice.org.uk/]

NHS Choice Framework. Information on conditions and healthy living for the public [https://www.gov.uk/government/publications/the-nhs-choice-framework/the-nhs-choice-framework-what-choices-are-available-to-me-in-the-nhs]

Nursing and Midwifery Council (NMC) [https://www.nmc.org.uk/]

Patient.info. One of the most trusted medical resources online, supplying evidence-based information on a wide range of medical and health topics to patients and health professionals [https://patient.info/]

Social Care Online. The UK's largest database of information and research on all aspects of social care and social work [https://www.scie.org.uk/social-care-online/]

WeNurses. X (formerly Twitter) based site that hosts 'chats' and has an 'X (formerly Twitter) versity' to help those new to X (formerly Twitter). Various professionals engage with this [http://www.wenurses.co.uk/]

Glossary

Abstract: A short summary of what a paper is about, usually printed at the beginning of the paper.

Accountable: To be answerable for your acts and your omissions.

Analysis: Breaking down a concept or an experience into parts.

Anecdotal evidence: Where personal opinion or information not based on proven facts is used as evidence.

Best available evidence: This is evidence that is found through a professional database search. It will depend on the question you are asking.

Campbell Collaboration: A worldwide collaboration that commissions and maintains systematic reviews in social care.

Case control study: A study in which people with a specific condition (cases) are compared with people without this condition (controls) to determine the frequency of occurrence of the exposure that might have caused the condition.

Cochrane Collaboration: A worldwide collaboration that commissions and maintains systematic reviews in health care.

Cohort study: A study in which two or more groups or cohorts are followed up to examine whether exposures measured at the beginning lead to outcomes, such as disease.

Confidence intervals: Confidence intervals are usually (but arbitrarily) 95 per cent confidence intervals. A reasonable, though strictly incorrect interpretation is that the 95 per cent confidence interval gives the range in which the population effect lies. A wide confidence interval implies a lack of certainty or precision about the true population effect and is commonly found in studies with too few participants.

Critical analysis: Where you break down or explore in depth all the information available relating to an issue or question. This may involve exploring what is happening and the reasons why. You may need to consider and access alternative perspectives including theory.

Critical appraisal: Where you consider the strengths and limitations of each piece of evidence you use.

Critical incident technique: When a significant incident is explored and analysed in order to improve decision-making and promote learning (see also **critical analysis**).

Critical thinking: Where you adopt a questioning approach and thoughtful attitude to what you read, see or hear, rather than accepting things at face value. It relates to both academic work and professional practice.

Database: A subject-specific database holds the references for, and often the abstracts or full text for, journal articles and many other texts, for which you can search using key words.

Debriefing: A structured facilitated approach often following stressful experiences. It can involve exploring coping strategies and lessons learned.

Description: Where information is given (verbally or in writing) in a factual manner.

Descriptive/narrative review: A review that is undertaken without a defined method. It is less likely to be comprehensive.

Descriptive statistics: Statistics such as means, medians and standard deviations that describe aspects of the data, such as central tendency (mean or median) or its dispersion (standard deviation).

Discussion paper: A paper presenting an argument or discussion.

Dissertation: A document presenting the method and the main findings from a piece of academic work.

Essay: A short piece of academic writing on a selected topic.

Ethnography: A qualitative research approach that involves the study of the culture or way of life of participants.

Evaluation: Judging and forming opinion, based on a sound argument – this involves the appraisal of information or evidence.

Evidence-based practice: Practice that is supported by clear reasoning, taking into account the patient's or client's preferences and using your own judgement.

Experiential knowledge: Knowledge gained by experience.

Experimental research: A study designed to test whether a treatment or intervention is effective.

Explanation: When using an explanatory style of writing or presenting, you provide justification or reasons for your actions, views and arguments.

Generalizability: Where the findings from a research study can be applied in other contexts.

Grounded theory: Qualitative research approach that involves the generation of theory.

Guideline: A systematically developed statement to assist practitioners in the delivery of evidence-based care.

Hierarchy of evidence: Strong evidence is at the top of the hierarchy and weaker evidence is at the bottom. Classifications as to what counts as strong evidence vary according to what you are endeavouring to find out.

Inferential statistics: Statistics that are used to infer findings from the sample population to the wider population, usually meaning statistical tests.

Inquisitive and open-minded: Aspects of critical thinking.

Intervention: An activity that intends to improve or effect health or social care outcomes.

Journal: An academic publication in which researchers publish their research.

Key words: Terms used when searching that represent the focus of the topic you wish to study.

Literature review: A collection of evidence on a particular topic (see **systematic review**).

Medical subject headings (MeSH): A thesaurus of medical terms used to index medical information in some databases.

Mixed methods research: Research that incorporates qualitative and quantitative research.

Narrative review: A literature review that is not undertaken according to a predefined and systematic approach.

Null hypothesis: A hypothesis stated in a neutral language, i.e. 'there is no difference between …'.

Open access journals: Journals that are freely available online rather than through an academic library.

p values: The p (probability) value is the probability of observing results more extreme than those observed if the null hypothesis were true.

Peer review: The process by which experts in a subject area are invited to review the academic work of an author, often prior to publication in a journal.

Phenomenology: Qualitative research approach in which the participants' 'lived experience' is explored.

PICOT: Acronym whose initials represent Population, Intervention/ Issue, Comparison/Context, Outcome and Time – sometimes shortened to **PICO.**

Professional judgement: The evaluation of information/evidence and the extent it is relevant to the care of your patients/clients. The end result of professional judgement is usually a decision.

Qualitative research: Generally uses interviews to explore the *experience* or *meaning* of an issue in depth. The results are presented as *words*.

Quantitative research: Generally used to explore if something is *effective or not*, or is used to measure the *amount of something*. The results are generally presented using *numbers* or *statistics*.

Questionnaires/surveys: Studies in which a sample is taken at *any one point in time* from *a defined group of people* and observed/assessed.

Randomization: The process of allocating individuals randomly to groups, usually in a randomized controlled trial.

Randomized controlled trial (RCT): A trial involving randomly assigned groups in order to determine the effectiveness of an intervention(s) given to one (or more) of the groups.

Rationale: Where you give clear reasons for your practice decisions or actions.

Readily available information: Information that you encounter on an everyday basis and do not need to look too hard for.

Reflection: Reflection is about reviewing an experience in order to learn from it.

Research: The systematic study developed from a research question to find out new knowledge.

Research question: A question set by researchers at the outset of a study, to be addressed in the study (see **PICOT**).

Research study/primary study: A study undertaken using a planned and methodological approach.

Reviews of research: see **Systematic review**.

Sample: The participants in a study.

Search strategy: A planned strategy to ensure a search is comprehensive.

Snowballing: A method of finding more literature by looking at the reference lists of papers you have found through a database search.

Student/learner: Any individual, pre- or post-qualifying, undertaking a course of study, either formally or informally.

Subject specific database: see **Database**.

Systematic review: A very detailed literature review that seeks to summarize all available evidence on a topic with clear explanations of the approach taken (methodology). It is the most detailed type of review.

Transferability: In qualitative studies, the findings may be used and interpreted by others, although the aim in qualitative research is not to generalize.

Truncation: The identification of a trunk of a word that is a stem for different words of similar meaning, e.g. nurs* (nurses/nursing/nurse).

References

All websites were accessible at the time of writing.

Alcock, P. and May, M. (2014) *Social Policy in Britain* (4th edition). Basingstoke: Palgrave Macmillan.

Atkins, S. and Schutz, S. (2013) Developing skills for reflective practice, in C. Bulman and S. Schutz (eds.) *Reflective Practice in Nursing* (5th edition). Oxford: Wiley-Blackwell.

Aveyard, H., Greenway, K. and Parsons, L. (2023) *A Beginner's Guide to Evidence Based Practice in Health and Social Care* (4th edition). Maidenhead: Open University Press.

Ayres, H. (2023) *The experiences of mental health nurses who have been assaulted by patients in medium secure mental health settings*. Thesis submitted for the award of a Professional Doctorate in Nursing, Oxford Brookes University.

Baldwin, A., Bentley, K., Langtree, T. and Mills, J. (2014) Achieving graduate outcomes in undergraduate nursing education: following the Yellow Brick Road, *Nurse Education in Practice*, 14 (1): 9–11.

Bandura, A. (1965) Influence of models' reinforcement contingencies on the acquisition of imitative responses, *Journal of Personality and Social Psychology*, 1 (6): 589–95.

Banning, M. (2008) A review of clinical decision making: models and current research, *Journal of Clinical Nursing*, 17 (2): 187–95.

Barnett, R. (1997) *Higher Education: A Critical Business*. Buckingham: SRHE/Open University Press.

Barnett, R. (2000) *Realizing the University in an Age of Supercomplexity*. Buckingham: SRHE/Open University Press.

Barnett, R. (2004) Learning for an unknown future, *Higher Education Research and Development*, 23 (3): 247–56.

Benner, P. (1984) *From Novice to Expert*. Menlo Park, CA: Addison-Wesley.

Blakemore, K. and Griggs, E. (2007) *Social Policy: An Introduction* (3rd edition). Maidenhead: Open University Press.

Bolton, G. (2010) *Reflective Practice: Writing and Professional Development* (3rd edition). London: Paul Chapman.

Bond, M. and Holland, S. (2010) *Skills of Clinical Supervision for Nurses: A Practical Guide for Supervisees, Clinical Supervisors and Managers* (Supervision in Context Series). Maidenhead: Open University Press.

Booth, S. (2010) Pregnant and can't give up smoking … despite son's pleas and risks to unborn baby, *Daily Record*, 29 June [http://www.dailyrecord.co.uk/news/real-life/pregnant-and-cant-give-up-smoking-1062988].

Bridges, D. (2000) Back to the future: the higher education curriculum in the twenty-first century, *Cambridge Journal of Education*, 30 (1): 37–55.

Brookfield, S. (2012) *Teaching for Critical Thinking: Tools and Techniques to Help Students Question Their Assumptions*. San Francisco, CA: Jossey-Bass.

Brotherton, G. and Parker, S. (2008) *Your Foundation in Health and Social Care*. London: Sage.

Brunt, B.A. (2005) Critical thinking in nursing: an integrated review, *Journal of Continuing Education in Nursing*, 36 (2): 60–67.

Bulman, C. and Schutz, S. (eds.) (2013) *Reflective Practice in Nursing* (5th edition). Oxford: Wiley-Blackwell.

Bulman, C. (2013a) An introduction to reflection, in C. Bulman and S. Schutz (eds.) *Reflective Practice in Nursing* (5th edition). Oxford: Wiley-Blackwell.

Bulman, C. (2013b) Getting started on a journey with reflection, in C. Bulman and S. Schutz (eds.) *Reflective Practice in Nursing* (5th edition). Oxford: Wiley-Blackwell.

Bulman, C., Lathlean, J. and Gobbi, M. (2012) The concept of reflection in nursing: qualitative findings on student and teacher perspectives, *Nurse Education Today*, 32 (5): e8–13 [https://doi.org/10.1016/j.nedt.2011.10.007].

Burnett, D. (2014) Hard to swallow: The world's first drinkable sunscreen, *The Guardian*, 20 May [http://www.theguardian.com/science/brain-flapping/2014/may/20/hard-to-swallow-the-worlds-first-drinkable-sunscreen].

Carter, B. (2013) Reflecting in groups, in C. Bulman and S. Schutz (eds.) *Reflective Practice in Nursing* (5th edition). Oxford: Wiley-Blackwell.

Catling, C., Davey, R., Donovan, H. and Dadich, A. (2024) A meta-synthesis of nurses and midwives' experience of clinical supervision, *Women and Birth*, 37 (1): 6-14 [https://doi.org/10.1016/j.wombi.2023.10.005].

Chatfield, T. (2018) *Critical Thinking: Your Guide to Effective Argument, Successful Analysis & Independent Study*. London: Sage.

Clarke, N. (2024) *The Student Nurses' Guide to Successful Reflection: Ten Essential Ingredients* (2nd edition). Open University Press. Maidenhead.

Cottrell, S. (2011) *Critical Thinking Skills: Developing Effective Argument and Analysis*. Basingstoke: Palgrave Macmillan.

Crawford, P., Brown, B., Kvangarsnes, M. and Gilbert, P. (2014) The design of compassionate care, *Journal of Clinical Nursing*, 23 (23/24): 3589–99.

Dahlgren, G. and Whitehead, M. (1993) *Policies and Strategies to Promote Health and Social Equity in Europe*. Stockholm: Institute of Futures Studies.

Dahlgren, G. and Whitehead, M. (2007) *European Strategies for Tackling Social Inequities in Health: Levelling Up Part 2*. Studies in Social and Economic Determinants of Population Health, No. 3. Copenhagen: WHO Regional Office for Europe [https://iris.who.int/bitstream/handle/10665/107791/E89384.pdf?sequence=1&isAllowed=y].

Deer, B. (2011) Secrets of the MMR scare: The *Lancet's* two days to bury bad news, *British Medical Journal*, 342: c7001 [https://doi.org/10.1136/bmj.c7001].

Delany, C., Golding, C. and Bialocerkowski, A. (2013) Teaching for thinking in clinical education: making explicit the thinking involved in allied health clinical reasoning, *Focus on Health Professional Education: A Multi-disciplinary Journal*, 14 (2): 44–56.

Demicheli, V., Rivetti, A., Debalini, M.G. and Di Pietrantonj, C. (2012) Vaccines for measles, mumps and rubella in children, *Cochrane Database of Systematic Reviews*, 2: CD004407 [https://doi.org/10.1002/14651858.CD004407.pub3].

Department of Health (DH) (2009) *Religion or Belief: A Practical Guide for the NHS*. London: DH [https://webarchive.nationalarchives.gov.uk/ukgwa/20130123195548/http:/www.dh.gov.uk/en/Publicationsandstatistics/Publications/PublicationsPolicyAndGuidance/DH_093133].

Driscoll, J. (2007) *Practising Clinical Supervision: A Reflective Approach for Healthcare Professionals*. Edinburgh: Baillière Tindall/Elsevier.

Dunphy, L., Proctor, G., Bartlett R., Haslam, M. and Wood, C. (2010) Reflections and learning from using action learning sets in a healthcare education setting, *Action Learning, Research and Practice*, 7 (3): 303–14.

Elliott, P. (2013) Moving from clinical supervision to person-centred development: a paradigm, in M. Jasper, M. Rosser and G. Mooney (eds.) *Professional Development, Reflection and Decision-Making in Nursing and Health Care* (2nd edition). Chichester: Wiley-Blackwell.

Elson, N., Le, D., Johnson, M., Reyna, C., Shaughnessy, E., Goodman, M. et al. (2021) Characteristics of general surgery social media influencers on Twitter, *American Surgeon*, 87(3): 492–98.

Facione, P.A. (1990) *Critical Thinking: A Statement of Expert Consensus for Purposes of Educational Assessment and Instruction. Executive Summary – 'The Delphi Report'*. Millbrae, CA: California Academic Press.

Facione, P.A. (2013) *Critical thinking: what it is and why it counts* [https://www.law.uh.edu/blakely/advocacy-survey/Critical%20Thinking%20Skills.pdf].

Fawcett, T.J.N., Rhynas, S.J. and Fawcett, T. (2014) Re-finding the 'human side' of human factors in nursing: helping student nurses to combine person-centred care with the rigours of patient safety, *Nurse Education Today*, 34 (9): 1238–41.

Felstead, I. (2013) Role modelling and students' professional development, *British Journal of Nursing*, 22 (4): 223–27.

Flanagan, J.C. (1954) The critical incident technique, *Psychological Bulletin*, 51 (4): 327–59.

Francis, R. (chair) (2013) *Report of the Mid Staffordshire NHS Foundation Trust Public Inquiry*. London: TSO [https://assets.publishing.service.gov.uk/media/5a7ba0faed915d13110607c8/0947.pdf].

Fraser, A.G. and Dunstan, F.D. (2010) On the impossibility of being expert, *British Medical Journal*, 341: c7126 [https://doi.org/10.1136/bmj.c6815].

Gallacher, J. and Osborne, M. (2005) *A Contested Landscape: International Perspectives on Diversity in Mass Higher Education*. Leicester: National Institute for Adult and Continuing Education.

Gibbs, G. (1988) *Learning by Doing: A Guide to Teaching and Learning Methods*. Oxford: Further Education Unit, Oxford Polytechnic.

Gillespie-Lynch, K., Hotez, E., Zajic, M., Riccio, A., DeNigris, D., Kofner, B. et al. (2020) Comparing the writing skills of autistic and nonautistic university students: a collaboration with autistic university students, *Autism*, 24 (7): 1898–912.

Goldacre, B. (2009) *Bad Science*. London: Harper Perennial.

Golding, C. (2011) Educating for critical thinking: thought-encouraging questions in a community of inquiry, *Higher Education Research & Development (Special Issue: Critical Thinking in Higher Education)*, 30 (3): 357–70.

Goleman, D., Boyatzis, R. and McKee, A. (2013) *Primal Leadership: Unleashing the Power of Emotional Intelligence.* Boston, MA: Harvard Business School Publishing.

Greenway, K. (2014) Rituals in nursing: intramuscular injections, *Journal of Clinical Nursing*, 23 (23/24): 3583–88.

Hargreaves, J. and Page, L. (2013) *Reflective Practice.* Cambridge: Polity Press.

Harrison, G. and Melville, R. (2010) *Rethinking Social Work in a Global World.* Basingstoke: Palgrave Macmillan.

Health and Care Professions Council (HCPC) (2012) *Standards of Conduct, Performance and Ethics.* London: HCPC (updated January 2016) [https://www.hcpc-uk.org/resources/standards/standards-of-conduct-performance-and-ethics/].

Health and Care Professions Council (HCPC) (2018) *Fitness to Practise – Raising Concerns.* London: HCPC [https://www.hcpc-uk.org.uk/concerns/raising-concerns/].

Health and Care Professions Council (HCPC) (2024) *Guidance on Social Media.* London: HCPC [https://www.hcpc-uk.org/globalassets/standards/standard-of-conduct-performance-and-ethics/revised-standards-2023/revised-guidance-on-social-media.pdf].

Held, D., McGrew, A., Goldblatt, D. and Perraton, J. (1999) *What is globalization?* [https://bcs.wiley.com/he-bcs/Books?action=mininav&bcsId=10913&itemId=074561499X&assetId=440967&resourceId=43093&newwindow=true].

Helms, M.M. and Nixon, J. (2010) Exploring SWOT analysis – where are we now? A review of academic research from the last decade, *Journal of Strategy and Management*, 3 (3): 215–51.

Holland, K. (2010) Culture, race and ethnicity: exploring the concepts, in K. Holland and C. Hogg, *Cultural Awareness in Nursing and Health Care: An Introductory Text* (2nd edition). London: Hodder Arnold.

Hosie, A., Agar, M., Lobb, E., Davidson, P.M. and Phillips, J. (2014) Palliative care nurses' recognition and assessment of patients with delirium symptoms: a qualitative study using critical incident technique, *International Journal of Nursing Studies*, 51 (10): 1353–65.

Huckabay, L.M. (2009) Clinical reasoned judgement and the nursing process, *Nursing Forum*, 44 (2): 72–78.

Jasper, M. (2013) *Beginning Reflective Practice* (2nd edition). Andover: Cengage Learning.

Jochemsen-van der Leeuw, R., van Dijk, N., van Etten-Jamaludin, F.S. and Wieringa-de Waard, M. (2013) The attributes of the clinical trainer as a role model: a systematic review, *Academic Medicine*, 88 (1): 26–34.

Johns, C. (2010) *Guided Reflection* (2nd edition). Oxford: Wiley-Blackwell.

Kedmey, D. (2014) Do mammograms save lives? 'Hardly', a new study finds, *Time Magazine*, 12 February [http://time.com/7117/do-mammograms-save-lives-hardly-a-new-study-finds/].

Keene, E.A., Hutton, N., Hall, B. and Ruston, C. (2010) Bereavement debriefing sessions: an intervention to support health care professionals in managing their grief after the death of a patient, *Pediatric Nursing*, 36 (4): 185–89.

Keogh, K. (2013) Nurses warned of disciplinary risk over improper Facebook postings, *Nursing Standard*, 27 (52): 7 [https://doi.org/10.7748/ns2013.08.27.52.7.s7].

Kida, T. (2006) *Don't Believe Everything You Think: The Six Basic Mistakes We Make in Thinking.* Amherst, NY: Prometheus Books.

Kotcher, J., Maibach, E., Miller, J., Campbell, E., Alqodmani, L., Maiero, M. et al. (2021) Views of health professionals on climate change and health: A multinational survey study, *The Lancet: Planetary Health*, 5: 5 [https://doi.org/10.1016/S2542-5196(21)00053-X].

Lang, G.M., Beach, N.L., Patrician, P.A. and Martin, C. (2013) A cross-sectional study examining factors related to critical thinking in nursing, *Journal for Nurses in Professional Development*, 29 (1): 8–15.

Leung, E.Y.L., Tirlapur, S.A., Siasssakos, D. and Khan, K.S. (2013) #BlueJC: *BJOG* and Katherine Twining Network collaborate to facilitate post-publication peer review and enhance research literacy via a Twitter journal club, *BJOG: An International Journal of Obstetrics and Gynaecology*, 120 (6): 657–60.

Levati, S. (2014) Professional conduct among Registered Nurses in the use of online social networking sites, *Journal of Advanced Nursing*, 70 (10): 2284–92.

Lovatt, A. (2014) Defining critical thoughts, *Nurse Education Today*, 34 (5): 670–72.

Luo, J., Du, J., Tao, C., Xu, H. and Zhang, Y. (2020) Exploring temporal suicide behaviour patterns on social media, *Health Information Journal*, 26 (2): 738–52.

Mann, K., Gordon, J. and MacLeod, A. (2009) Reflection and reflective practice in health professions: a systematic review, *Advances in Health Science Education*, 14 (4): 595–621.

McCormack, B., Kim Manley, K. and Titchen, A. (eds.) (2013) *Practice Development in Nursing and Healthcare* (2nd edition). Oxford: Wiley.

Miller, A.B., Wall, C., Baines, C.J., Sun, P., To, T. and Narod, S.A. (2014) Twenty five year follow-up for breast cancer incidence and mortality of the Canadian National Breast Screening Study: randomised screening trial, *British Medical Journal*, 348: g366 [https://doi.org/10.1136/bmj.g366].

Nursing and Midwifery Council (NMC) (2010) Annexe 3: Essential skills clusters (2010) and guidance for their use (guidance G7.1.5b), in *Standards for Pre-registration Nursing Education* [https://www.nmc.org.uk/globalassets/sitedocuments/standards/nmc-standards-for-pre-registration-nursing-education.pdf].

Nursing and Midwifery Council (NMC) (2018) *The Code: Professional Standards of Practice and Behaviour for Nurses, Midwives and Nursing Associates*. London: NMC [https://www.nmc.org.uk/globalassets/sitedocuments/nmc-publications/nmc-code.pdf].

Nursing and Midwifery Council (NMC) (2023a) *Guidance on Using Social Media Responsibly*. London: NMC [https://www.nmc.org.uk/standards/guidance/social-media-guidance/].

Nursing and Midwifery Council (NMC) (2023b) *Raising Concerns: Guidance for Nurses, Midwives and Nursing Associates*. London: NMC [https://www.nmc.org.uk/standards/guidance/raising-concerns-guidance-for-nurses-and-midwives/].

Office for National Statistics (ONS) (2022) *Population and Household Estimates, England and Wales: Census 2021*, ONS Statistical Bulletin [https://www.ons.gov.uk/peoplepopulationandcommunity/populationandmigration/populationestimates/bulletins/populationandhouseholdestimatesenglandandwales/census2021unroundeddata#cite-this-statistical-bulletin].

Oozageer Gunowa, N., Hutchinson, M., Brooke, J., Aveyard, H., and Jackson, D. (2021). Pressure injuries and skin tone diversity in undergraduate nurse education: Qualitative perspectives from a mixed methods study. *Journal of Advanced Nursing*, 77 (11): 4511–24.

Paul, R. and Elder, L. (2005) *Critical Thinking: Tools for Taking Charge of Your Professional and Personal Life*. Upper Saddle River, NJ: Prentice-Hall.

Paul, R. and Elder, L. (2014) *Critical Thinking: Tools for Taking Charge of Your Professional and Personal Life* (2nd edition). Boston, MA: Pearson Education.

Perry, B. (2009) Role modelling excellence in clinical nursing practice, *Nurse Education in Practice*, 9 (1): 36–44.

Pertwee, E., Simas, C. and Larson, C. (2022) An epidemic of uncertainty, *Nature Medicine*, 28: 456–59.

Price, B. and Harrington, A. (2019) *Critical Thinking and Writing in Nursing* (4th edition). Exeter: Learning Matters.

Ramondt, S., Zijlska, M., Kerkhof, P. and Merz, E. (2020) Barriers to blood donation on social media: an analysis of Facebook and Twitter posts, *Transfusion*, 60 (10): 2294–306.

Reid, B. (1993) 'But we're doing it already': exploring a response to the concept of reflective practice in order to improve its facilitation, *Nurse Education Today*, 13 (4): 305–9.

Roberts, D. (2013) *Psychosocial Nursing Care: A Guide to Nursing the Whole Person*. Maidenhead: Open University Press.

Romanello, M., di Napoli, C., Green, C., Kennard, H., Lampard, P., Scamman, D. et al. (2023) The 2023 report of the Lancet Countdown on health and climate change: the imperative for a health-centred response in a world facing irreversible harms, *The Lancet*, 402 (10419): 2346–94

Royal College of Nursing (RCN) (2019) *RCN Position Statement: Responding to Climate Change* [https://www.rcn.org.uk/Professional-Development/publications/pub-007878].

Rutter, L. and Brown, K. (2020) *Critical Thinking and Professional Judgement for Social Work* (5th edition). London: Sage.

Seedhouse, D. (2009) *Ethics: The Heart of Healthcare* (3rd edition). Chichester: Wiley.

Sicora, A., Taylor, B., Alfandari, R., Enosh, G., Helm, D., Killick, C. et al. (2021) Using intuition in social work decision making, *European Journal of Social Work*, 24 (5): 772–87.

Simone, B., Carrillo-Santisteve, P. and Lopalco, P.L. (2012) Healthcare workers' role in keeping MMR vaccination uptake high in Europe, *Eurosurveillance*, 17 (26): 20206 [https://www.eurosurveillance.org/images/dynamic/EE/V17N26/art20206.pdf].

Smith, G.C.S. and Pell, J.P. (2003) Parachute use to prevent death and major trauma related to gravitational challenge: systematic review of randomised controlled trials, *British Medical Journal*, 327 (7429): 1459–61.

Smith, R. (2010) Strategies for coping with information overload, *British Medical Journal*, 341: c7126 [https://doi.org/10.1136/bmj.c7126].

Social Care Institute for Excellence (SCIE) (2008) *Learning Organisations: A Self-Assessment Resource Pack*. London: SCIE.

Stacey, T., Samples, J., Leadley, C., Alcester, L. and Jenney, A. (2022) 'I don't need you to criticize me, I need you to support me': a qualitative study of women's experiences of and attitudes to smoking cessation, *Women and Birth*, 35 (6): e549–55.

Standing, M. (2011) *Clinical Judgement and Decision Making for Nursing Students.* Exeter: Learning Matters.

Stillwell, S.B., Finehout-Overholt, E., Mazurek, B. and Williamson, K. (2010) Evidence-based practice, step by step. Asking the clinical question: a key step in evidence-based practice, *American Journal of Nursing*, 110 (3): 58–61.

Tate, S. (2013) Writing to learn: writing reflectively, in C. Bulman and S. Schutz (eds.) *Reflective Practice in Nursing* (5th edition). Oxford: Wiley-Blackwell.

Thompson, C., Aitken, L., Doran, D. and Dowding, D. (2013) An agenda for clinical decision making and judgement in nursing research and education, *International Journal of Nursing Studies*, 50 (12): 1720–26.

Tripp, D. (2011) *Critical Incidents in Teaching: Developing Professional Judgement* (classic edition). London: Routledge.

United Nations (1987) *Report of the World Commission on Environment and Development.* General Assembly Resolution 42/187, 9th Plenary Meeting,11 December 1987 [https://digitallibrary.un.org/record/153026?ln=en&v=pdf].

United Nations (2009) *World Population Ageing – 2009* [https://www.un.org/esa/socdev/documents/ageing/Data/WorldPopulationAgeingReport2009.pdf].

United Nations (undated) *What are the Sustainable Development Goals?* [https://www.undp.org/sustainable-development-goals].

United Nations Environment Programme/World Health Organization (UNEP/WHO) (2008) *Libreville Declaration on Health and Environment in Africa.* Libreville, Gabon: WHO Regional Office for Africa [https://www.afro.who.int/publications/libreville-declaration].

Vachon, B. and LeBlanc, J. (2011) Effectiveness of past and current critical incident analysis on reflective learning and practice change, *Medical Education*, 45 (9): 894–904.

Wakefield, A.J., Murch, S.H., Anthony, A. and Linnell, J. (1998) Ileal-lymphoid-nodular hyperplasia, non-specific colitis and pervasive developmental disorder in children, *The Lancet*, 351 (9103): 637–41 (article retracted).

Wallace, M. and Wray, A. (2016) *Critical Reading and Writing for Postgraduates* (3rd edition). London: Sage.

Walter, P. and Owens, R.J.Q. (2013) *How to Study in College* (11th edition). Andover: Cengage Learning.

Watson, G. and Glaser, E. (2012) *Watson-Glaser Critical Thinking Appraisal – User Guide and Technical Manual*. London: Pearson Education.

Wellington, J., Bathmaker, A., Hunt, C., McCulloch, G. and Sikes P. (2005) *Succeeding with Your Doctorate*. London: Sage.

Wolf, Z.R. (2014) *Exploring Rituals in Nursing*. New York: Springer.

Woolliams, M., Williams, K., Butcher, D. and Pye, D. (2009) *Be More Critical! A Practical Guide for Health and Social Care Students*. Oxford: Oxford Brookes University.

World Health Organization (WHO) (2006) *Constitution of the World Health Organization*. Geneva: WHO [https://www.who.int/publications/m/item/constitution-of-the-world-health-organization].

World Health Organization (WHO) (2008) *mhGAP: Mental Health Gap Action Programme: Scaling Up Care for Mental, Neurological, and Substance Use Disorders*. Geneva: WHO [https://www.who.int/publications/i/item/9789241596206].

World Health Organization (WHO) (2011) *10 Facts on Preventing Disease from Healthy Environments*. Geneva: WHO.

World Health Organization (WHO) (2014) *Malaria*. Fact sheet No. 94. Geneva: WHO [https://reliefweb.int/report/world/malaria-fact-sheet-no-94-updated-march-2014].

Zegeye, B., Ahinkorah, B., Ameyaw, E., Budu, E., Abdul-Aziz, S., Comfort, Z. et al. (2022) Disparities in use of skilled birth attendants and neonatal mortality in Guinea over two decades, *BMC Pregnancy and Childbirth*, 22: 56 [https://doi.org/10.1186/s12884-021-04370-8].

Index

Page numbers in italics are figures.

abstracts 54
accountability 21–2
action learning sets 129
advice 27, 32–3
aims *see* research questions
analysis, style of writing 96–7, 98
anecdotal evidence 19, 60, 61
appraisal/analysis 90–1
assessment
  of alternatives 119–20
  self- 122–3, 125
assignments, academic 23–5
assumptions, challenging 6
Atkins, S. 125
Ayres, H. 152

Baldwin, A. 120
Bandura, A. 120
Barnett, R. 123
best available evidence 43–5, 55–8,
  75
  demonstrating use of 89
  research evidence 58–62
    qualitative 59, 60, 61, 62–4, 70–3
    quantitative 59, 60, 64–73
  search process for 45–6
  subject-specific electronic
    databases 46–9
  up-to-date research 73–4
bias 2, 30, 38, 39
blogs 32
Bond, M. 128
Boolean operators 51
broadening horizons 160–70
Brookfield, S. 6, 120–1, 136, 147–8

Brotherton, G. 130
Brown, K. 3, 4
Bulman, C. 97, 124, 127–8, 130

Campbell Collaboration 37–8, 56
Carter, B. 129
case control studies 65
challenging practice 133–6, *134*
changes in health and social care
  148–55, 170
  broadening horizons 160–70
  critical thinking response 156–7,
    156
  skills and qualities 158–60
Chatfield, T. 6
CINAHL 19
citing information 15
Clarke, N. 125
climate change 154–5
Cochrane Collaboration 37–8, 56
cohort studies 65
communication technology 149–50
conference presentations 34–5
confidence intervals 68–9
coping strategies 158
Cornell note-taking system 84–5, *84*
COVID-19 7, 18, 32, 33, 153
creativity 158
critical analysis 13, 15, 131
critical appraisal 9, 13, 90, 96, 105,
  107
Critical Appraisal Skills Programme
  (CASP) 64, 70
critical being 123
critical friends 127–8

critical incident analysis (CIA) 130
critical thinking, defining 5–9, 10

Dahlgren, G. 156–7, *156*
data collection
    qualitative research 63–4
    quantitative research 66–70
databases 18–19, 45
    planning searches 49–54
    subject-specific 46–9
debriefing 130
Delany, C. 136–7
descriptive reviews 38, 57–8
descriptive statistics 66–7
descriptive writing 94, 98
diaries, reflective 127, 128
discussion papers 39
diversity of populations 150–1
documenting search strategies 52–3
Driscoll, J. 126, *126*
Dunphy, L. 129

e-books 35–6, 54
editorials 37
Elder, L. 123
electronic journals 36
environmental issues 154–5
escalating concerns 135–6
ethnography 63
evaluation, style of writing 95, 98
evidence
    objective 4
    for professional practice 132–6,
        134
    see also information/evidence
evidence-based knowledge
        summaries 39–41
evidence-based practice 17–18, 119
experience
    personal 4–5, 146–8
    and professional practice 119–20
explanation style of writing 94, 98

Facione, P.A. 5, 10, 11, 122–3, 123
Felstead, I. 33, 121
financial resources 152
Flanagan, J.C. 130

flexibility 148, 158
focus, in writing and presentations
        86–7
focus groups 63–4
Francis, R. 112

generalisability 66, 69
Glaser, E. 123
globalization 155
Goldacre, Ben 9
Goleman, D. 125
Google 45–6
Greenway, K. 118
grounded theory 62
guidance, professional and clinical
        39–41, 136

hard copy 36
Hargreaves, J. 124
Harrington, A. 5, 112
Health and Care Professions Council
        (HCPC) 21, 32, 113, 136, 151
hierarchy of evidence 55, 59–62
history of critical thinking 7, 7–8
Holland, S. 128

importance of critical thinking 2–5,
        5, 145–8
inequalities, health 152–3
inferential statistics 67–8, 70
influences, life 146–8
information overload 18–23
information/evidence 26–7
        categories 14
        readily available 27–8
interest groups 163–4
internet searches 27, 29
interviews 63–4

Jochemsen-van der Leeuw, R. 120
Johns, C. 127
journals 27, 37–41, *39*, 41, 54
        electronic 36
        learning 127

Keene, E.A. 130
key words 49, 50, 51–2

Kida, T. 4
knowledge management 18–23
Kotcher, J. 155

lack of critical thinking 3, 4, 7–8
Lang, G.M. 119
language, in writing and
    presentations 87–8
law *see* legal responsibilities
leaflets 27–8
LeBlanc, J. 130
lectures/lecture notes 27, 34–5
legal responsibilities 22–3
literature reviews 55–6, 57–8
Lovatt, A. 120

McCormack, B. 118
mammography example 10–12
Manchester Academic Phrase
    Bank 89
Mann, K. 124, 127
marking systems 23, 83
media *see* newspapers/news
    websites; social media
meta-commentary 88–9
mind maps 85–6, *85*
mixed methods studies 59

narrative reviews 57–8
networking 150, 160, 163–5
newspapers/news websites 27, 28–9
null hypothesis 69
Nursing and Midwifery Council
    (NMC) 21, 32, 113, 136, 151

Oozageer Gunowa, N. 151
opinion papers 39
'ostrich strategy' 19–20

p values 68–9
Page, L. 124
Parker, S. 130
patients/clients (term) xviii
Paul, R. 123
Pell, J.P. 74
person-centred care 112, 131,
    139–40

person-centred development 128–9
Pertwee, E. 7, 18
phenomenology 62–3
PICOT 49–50
'pigeon strategy' 20
plagiarism 89
policy 14, 39–41
    changes in 153–4
politics 153–4
populations, diversity of 150–1
practice, professional *see*
    professional practice
presentations
    verbal 77–8, 79, 105–7, *107*, 109
        approach to 86–92
        checklist 107–8
        developing 80–1
        planning to 81–6, *82*
        styles 92–8
Price, B. 5, 112
professional bodies 112–13, 163–4
professional judgement 13, 18,
    119–20
professional knowledge 17, 20
professional practice 23–5, 110–13,
    142, 165–70
    assessing development skills
      122–3
    development 131–2
    evidence 132–6, *134*
    and experience 119–20
    influencing critical thinking
      culture 141–2
    and professional bodies 112–13
    questions for in-depth approach
      136–41
    reflection 123–31, *126*
    and routine 114–19

qualitative research 59, 60, 61, 62–4
    examples 70–3
quality of information 15
quantitative research 59, 60, 64–70
    examples 70–3
quasi experiments 65
questioning/challenging practice of
    others 133–6, *134*

questionnaires 65–6
questions for critical thinking 12–15, *16*, 136–9
quotes from authors 89

rainbow model 156–7, *156*
raising concerns 135–6
randomised control trials (RCTs) 60, 61, 65
readily available information 27–8, 41
  advice 32–3
  hard copy and electronic journals 36
  internet sources/general search engines 29
  lectures/conference presentations 34–5
  newspaper/news websites 28–9
  social media 31–2
  textbooks/e-books 35–6
  websites 29–31
reflection 3, 123–31, *126*
  style of writing 97, 98
reflective frameworks 126–7, *126*
research 14
research evidence/studies 58–9
  types 59–62
Research Gate 54
research questions 38, 58–9, 62, 64–5, 72–3
research studies 38–9, *39*
resources, financial/material 152
responsibilities 22–3
responsiveness 158
reviews of research 19
rituals, in nursing 117–18
role models 120–2
Romanello, M. 155
routine 114–19
Rutter, L. 3, 4

Schutz, S. 125, 130
search engines 29, 45–6
self-assessment
  and self-awareness 125
  tools 122–3

self-awareness 125–6
Simone, B. 9
six questions for critical thinking 12–15, *16*
Smith, G.C.S. 74
Smith, R. 19–20
Social Care Institute for Excellence 141
social determinants of health model 156–7, *156*
social media 27, 31–2, 150
social wellbeing inequalities 152–3
sources
  conflicting 9–12
  see also readily available information
spider diagrams 85–6, *85*
Standing, M. 120
structure, in writing and presentations 87–8
summaries, knowledge 39–40
summarizing 91–2
supervision, professional/clinical 128–9
surveys 65–6
Sustainable Development Goals (SDGs) (UN) 153
SWOT analysis tool 131–2
synthesis 91
systematic reviews 37–8, 55, 56–7, 60, 61

Tate, S. 127
technology
  communication 149–50
  internet searches 27, 29, 53
terms used xviii
textbooks 27, 35–6
theory 14
Thompson, C. 119–20
transferability 63
truncation facility 51
Twitter *see* X (formerly Twitter)

Vachon, B. 130
viewpoints, alternative 91

Wallace, M. 14
Watson, G. 123
websites 27, 29–31
Wellington, J. 80–1
'What?' model 126, *126*
Whitehead, M. 156–7, *156*
Wolf, Z.R. 117–18
Woolliams, M. 14, 16
World Health Organization (WHO 2011) 154–5
Wray, A. 14

writing 77–9, 109
    approach to 86–92
    checklist 107–8
    developing 80–1
    example 98–105
    planning the work 81–6, *82*
    styles 92–8

X (formerly Twitter) 31–2

Zegeye, B. 67–9